ESSENTIAL BEAUTY

ESSENTIAL 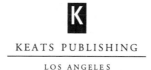BEAUTY

USING NATURE'S ESSENTIAL OILS TO REJUVENATE, REPLENISH, AND REVITALIZE

PATRICIA BETTY

with David Andrusia

K

KEATS PUBLISHING

LOS ANGELES

NTC/Contemporary Publishing Group

Library of Congress Cataloging-in-Publication Data

Betty, Patricia.
    Essential beauty : using nature's essential oils to rejuvenate, replenish,
    and revitalize / Patricia Betty, with David Andrusia.
        p. cm.
    Includes bibliographical references and index.
    ISBN 0-658-00280-5
        1. Skin—Care and hygiene. 2. Aromatherapy. 3. Essences and
    essential oils. I. Andrusia, David. II. Title.

    RL87.B48 2000
    646.7'26—dc21
                                                            00-020326

Published by Keats Publishing
A division of NTC/Contemporary Publishing Group, Inc.
4255 West Touhy Avenue, Lincolnwood, Illinois 60646-1975 U.S.A.

Design by Laurie Young
Frontispiece illustration by Carol Hamoy
Interior illustrations by Ilene Robinette

Printed in the United States of America

International Standard Book Number: 0-658-00280-5

00 01 02 03 04 DHD 18 17 16 15 14 13 12 11 10 9 8 7 6 5 4 3 2 1

To all our fellow travelers

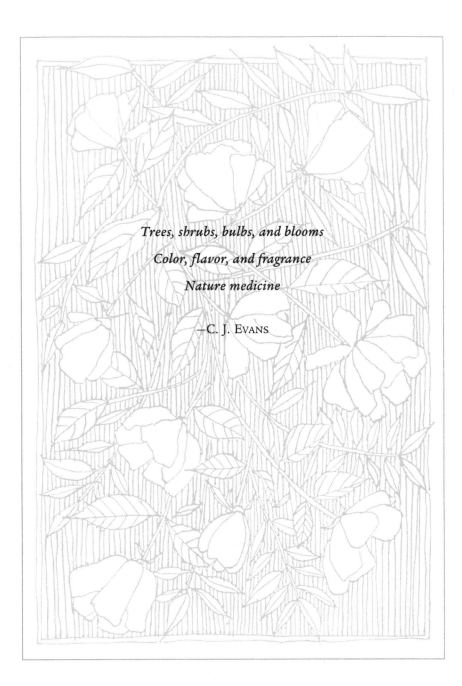

Trees, shrubs, bulbs, and blooms

Color, flavor, and fragrance

Nature medicine

—C. J. EVANS

CONTENTS

ACKNOWLEDGMENTS

Thanks to my wonderful clients and students for their valuable feedback and prodding; to Marie Zazzi for just being; to Maureen Ressler of Elizabeth Arden for her support and loyalty; to the teachers and staff of the New York Botanical Garden; to Peter Hoffman for his gentleness and commitment to this book; to David Andrusia for suggesting this book and making it happen; and to our editor, Phyllis Herman, who pulled it all together.

—PATRICIA BETTY

Thanks to Pat Betty for friendship, wonderful Jamaican patties, and even more wonderful skin; to Peter Hoffman for believing in this book; to Greg Ptacek for introducing me to Peter; and to Phyllis Herman for making this the best book it could be.

—DAVID ANDRUSIA

INTRODUCTION

PERHAPS THE QUESTION I AM ASKED MOST OFTEN IS THIS: HOW DID someone with a degree in cell biology become an aromatherapist and alternative health practitioner?

Like most passions, my love of plants and their oils began in childhood. As a youngster, I attended a wonderful girls' school in Kingston, Jamaica, where students were encouraged to study a variety of subjects and to learn for enjoyment's sake. From as early as I can remember, my favorite subjects were biology, botany, health science, gourmet cooking, and literature.

Of course, the fact that I was growing up in what was (at the time) one of the most beautiful and unspoiled areas in the world helped to color my view of the world. My environment also added spice to my observations and interpretations of the world.

How could I not love nature when I was surrounded by the brilliant hues and contrasts of nature at her flamboyant best? How could I not love beautifully prepared and presented foods, when I had always had at my fingertips a mouthwatering display of spices, herbs, and oils with which to creatively enhance fresh foods? Together, all these turned family mealtimes into unforgettable taste sensations.

As I grew older, how could I not love the wondrous, life-affirming scents of essential oils when introduced to aromatherapy? After all, I had been raised to absorb the perfumes of the tropics both subconsciously and consciously. These included hypnotically sweet flowers with a citrus overlay, deepened with ripening fruits like mangoes and pineapples, spices, and coffee, all of which wafted over the island thanks to the ever-present ocean breezes and mountain rain. So my senses were already tuned up, waiting to absorb the beautiful complexities of aromatherapy.

Ever after, I have come to view good health and beauty as an incorporation of good food lovingly prepared, good habits, an appreciation of nature's bounty, and a joyous and open mind. Nothing I have seen throughout life has changed this view.

How did I choose a career in aromatherapy? My sister, who lived in London, sent me articles about this oddly named "new" alternative treatment. Although she herself was mystified by its popularity, she was sure it was something that I, who had always explored uncharted paths, would be interested in. Meanwhile, my other sister had already sent me masses of literature about physical and beauty therapy schools in England. Something clicked: This was a chance to combine research on well-being with actual hands-on practice. I found a highly respected beauty therapy institute that catered to my intellectual and professional needs, moved to London practically overnight—and the rest, as they say, is history!

Following my initial training in aroma- and beauty therapy, I expanded my studies to include cell biology, genetics, and botany at Lesley College in Cambridge, Massachusetts. I studied acupressure with Dr. Stephen Chang at the Acupressure Center for Chinese Medicine, and medical massage therapy at the Swedish Institute for Massage Therapy in New York City, along with other related studies.

When I first started working on clients with the massage and aromatherapy techniques I had developed, choosing the best of the many modalities I had studied while observing the reactions of my clients, I soon began to notice a radiant glow on their faces as the treatment progressed. In fact, many of my neediest clients actually seemed to be reborn! Clients often come in looking gray and frazzled, but two hours later, they leave with rosy cheeks, sparkling eyes, and a visible lightness of being. When I worked on dancers at the School for Creative Movement in New York City, the owners began to recognize my clients by that very radiance. So much so, in fact, that they'd ask dancers who looked absolutely revitalized, "You look sensational. . . . Have you just been Pat Betty-ized?"

Years of experience and experimentation have gone into my formulas and treatments. Since my interest in health, beauty, and the restorative properties of plants dates back to early childhood, I have long experimented on myself and (often fairly unwilling!) childhood friends and family members, using the wildly exotic plant masks I'd devised myself. Gradually, I came to understand that you could actually reprogram skin cells by using essential plant oils both internally, when eaten as part of a healthy diet, and externally, when applied to the skin. The combination results in beauty boosters that are second to none.

Combining existing research, my own trials, and my knowledge of biology and cell life, I developed the aromatherapeutic facials I now offer to clients in New York and around the world. Some of my clients look as if they've just had a face-lift after they've left my office! In truth, all of them have a newfound glow, thanks to the natural bounty of essential oils and plant extracts.

And now, so can you! Whatever your skin color or complexion type, and even if your skin is supersensitive, you can glow with inner and outer beauty, thanks to the array of oils and programs I'll introduce you to in the chapters that follow.

Your first day of a healthy new beauty is today!

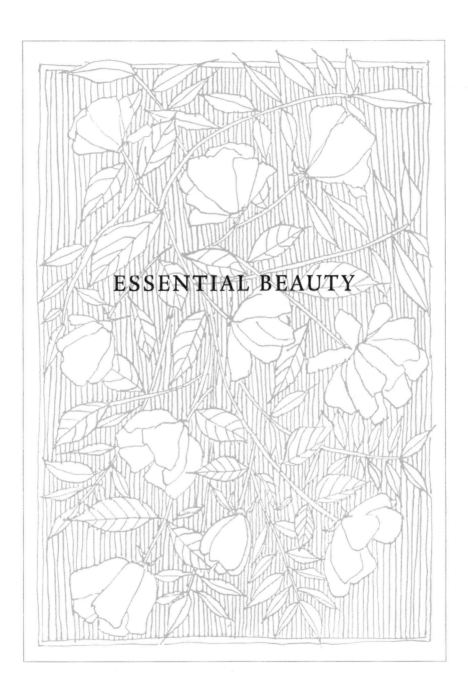

ESSENTIAL BEAUTY

CHAPTER 1

WHAT ARE ESSENTIAL OILS?

ESSENTIAL OILS ARE STRONGLY SCENTED FRAGRANT MOLECULES FOUND in different parts of a variety of plants. Although there are many different fragrances found in nature, aromatherapists define essential oils as the scented molecules comprised mainly of compound chemicals called terpenes. Plants create terpenes during pollination, as a means of self-protection, for hydration, and to implement boundary control, among other reasons. Terpenes contain important medicinal compounds and cosmetic ingredients. Interestingly, essential oils are self-preserving: They never "die," but they do evaporate, and they can be changed structurally by overexposure to light, heat, and water. We get essential oils from relatively few plants, but they cover a variety of plant species and they come from nearly all parts of a plant. Essential oils can be derived from flower petals (as in the rose); leaves (eucalyptus, cypress, bay); seeds (coriander, fennel, carrot); roots (vetiver, ginger); herbs (melissa, peppermint, sage); fruit skins (orange, lemon); and other parts of the plant as well.

WHAT *AREN'T* ESSENTIAL OILS?

There's a lot of confusion about essential oils, especially since huge product manufacturers have recently tried to appropriate aromatherapy for themselves. More times than not, the "herbal essence" shampoo you buy claims to contain "essential oils," but these oils are often manufactured in a laboratory in New Jersey; they are not the essences of plants from exotic places around the world. Their product descriptions are merely capitalizing on the popularity of aromatherapy.

These ersatz herbal products might smell nice (though I assure you that their scents are nothing compared to those of real essential oils), but their professed powers are almost always figments of a marketer's imagination. These manufactured molecules are mostly synthetic. Since they possess none of a real essential oil's natural properties, they possess none of their benefits either.

HOW ARE ESSENTIAL OILS EXTRACTED?

The overwhelming majority of essential oils are extracted by the process of steam distillation. This is a very efficient and relatively inexpensive way to process many leaves, seeds, woods, and root oils.

In addition, some petals—principally those of rose, lavender, chamomile, and orange blossom (neroli)—are also processed by the distillation method, and the water remaining at the end of the processing is bottled and sold as floral water or hydrolats. These floral waters are used in a variety of ways. Rose and neroli are sometimes used in gourmet desserts, and all the floral waters are excellent as skin toners, air fresheners, and after-bath splashes.

Another method of extraction is maceration. This process is most often used to obtain the essential oils from the peels of citrus fruits.

Enfleurage is a fat-based extraction process in which parts of plants (usually flower petals) are laid out on trays smeared with oil. In time, the essential oils from the petals will leach out into the carrier oil. This method is an updated and refined version of the oil infusion method, which was used by the ancients and to some extent is still used today, for example, in herb-infused salad oils.

Chemical solvent extraction was developed by perfumers and traditionally has been used for hard-to-extract flowers. The resulting "absolute" has many deep and tantalizing tones that have long been valued by perfumers. Interestingly, some aromatherapy purists prefer not to use absolutes because they are afraid the essential oils may be tainted by the solvent. However, I am convinced that the essential oils will always rise above their surroundings. For this reason, I have been using absolutes with confidence in my practice for the last eighteen years. They are very expensive, but happily, a little goes a long way!

In addition to these medicinal properties, essential oils also contain such natural health and beauty aids as:

- vitamins
- minerals
- amino acids
- oxygen
- humectants
- pH balancers
- firming agents
- detoxifiers

HOW ARE ESSENTIAL OILS USED?

Essential oil therapy, also called aromatherapy, has been with us in one form or another since ancient times. In fact, our early ancestors clearly recognized the superiority and uniqueness of scented plants. So powerful and pungent were the scents emanating from these plants that humans quickly developed a communication with them and practiced traditions that still exist today.

The two major traditions that date back to people's first relationship with plants are esoteric rituals and life support uses.

THE MEDICINAL PROPERTIES OF ESSENTIAL OILS

Function	Action	Essential Oils
Analgesic	Pain-reducing	Allspice, bay, birch, clove, basil, peppermint, pennyroyal, eucalyptus
Antihistamine	Provides relief from allergic reactions	Eucalyptus, lavender, basil, peppermint, spearmint, pennyroyal
Anti-inflammatory	Relieves inflammation	Bay, birch, benzoin, basil, clove, lavender, lemon, peppermint, eucalyptus, spearmint, nutmeg, and others
Antioxidant	Slows the rate of oxidation in the body through the actions of such phytonutrients as rutin, rosemarinic acid, eugenol, coumaric acid, and vanillic acid	All essential oils
Circulation booster	Keeps circulation moving freely	Most, but especially geranium
Diuretic	Helps release excess water from the system	All essential oils
Expectorant	Removes mucus from the system	Peppermint, eucalyptus, ginger, basil, frankincense, thyme, spearmint

Out of the esoteric rituals evolved many beautiful and poetic forms of "journeying," a communication between humans and higher, invisible powers. This tradition manifests itself today in such rituals as the burning of incense in churches and temples, the spice box used in the Jewish Habdalah service marking the end of the Sabbath, and the tradition of some West African–based religions that use scented oils as anointing agents. Native civilizations around the world continue to base their religions—indeed, their entire cultural lives—on various forms of journeying.

The life support uses were centered around the use of plants on the human body, as well as to enhance food and drink. I call this "quality of life" usage. These plants can enhance our lives from cradle to grave (and even beyond), according to many ancient traditions. We can use them for grooming, as medicines, to aid with birthing, as aphrodisiacs, to celebrate weddings, and to see our beloved deceased off to the next world. Plants and their essences had and still have a place in virtually every important aspect of life.

ESSENTIAL OILS AND
YOUR SENSE OF SMELL

The overwhelming majority of my friends and clients immediately fall in love with the ethereal and earthy scents of essential oils, as I did upon first encountering them some twenty years ago. So inundated are we with manufactured, artificial scents that we sometimes forget how marvelous those of nature can be!

Once in a while, a new client will complain that essential oils smell "too strong." People who have been overexposed to toxins; those who eat mainly processed, overly salted, fried fast foods or drink too much beer; and those who are used to overly processed synthetic fragrances and perfumes may be turned off by the smell of real essential oils. It is unfortunate that our unhealthy modern-day diet and environment have dulled and distorted our scent sensitivity. Aromatherapy can help. Starting an aromatherapeutic beauty regimen is the perfect time to improve our diet and reacquaint ourselves with our God-given sense of smell.

By far the most important distortion of our scent receptors is a result of the distortion of our taste buds. Innately, we humans are able to taste sweet, sour, salty, bitter, and a complex subtle array of other flavors, by way of chemical sense perceptors and scent receptors in the nose and tongue. However, if we kill these subtle receptors by eating too much salt, fat, or refined sugar, we lose the ability not only to taste but to smell. Rather than appreciating nature's own exquisite nuances, aromas, and flavors, we can only perceive the harshest, grossest, and strongest ones—the supersalty, the supersugary, and the supersweet "fragrances" department stores sell.

Thus, our senses of taste and smell are inextricably intertwined. If we can't taste properly, we can't smell properly, either, because our mucous membranes are not allowing free movement and are blocked in other areas as well. That is why people with digestive or lung congestion often sound as if they have a head cold when they speak. More often than not, these folks breathe through their mouths because of the nasal passageway blockage, thus worsening their perceptions of smell and taste.

By using the food and beauty plans presented in the following chapters, you will be virtually readjusting your system. Then you can truly get in touch with the natural goodness of the Earth's bountiful foods and scents.

THE MIND/BODY/SPIRIT/ EMOTION CONNECTION

Nowhere is the mind/body/spirit/emotion connection more dramatic than in aromatherapy. Essential oils dramatically uplift the spirits even while they are clearing the mind, cleansing the body, and balancing the emotions. When you massage an aromatherapy blend into your face, you immediately see and feel a remarkable difference. That difference shows itself in a rush of circulation to the skin and a fresher, more radiant look—plus, best of all, a softer, silkier feel to the skin.

Aromatherapy creams, lotions, and ampules all contribute to wonderful skin health. My preference, however, is to use blended essential oils in a vegetable oil base. I find that when these aromatherapeutic oils are mixed with this carrier base, they interact more dramatically with the skin to produce a radiance that mere creams can't match.

In this country, many people (and even some practitioners) are biased against the use of oils because they fear oils will leave the skin feeling greasy and clogged. This is decidedly not the case—indeed, the skin *loves* aromatherapy oils and shows its appreciation at once. You can also notice the oils' positive effect by the heat generated on the skin while you are massaging them in. Creams and lotions, even those with essential oils mixed in, remain cool (even cold) to the touch. Their vibrations are more sluggish and are not easily speeded up by the essential oils (which themselves vibrate at incredibly fast rates). Vegetable oils, on the other hand, respond immediately to the prodding of essential oils by becoming warm and silky to the touch as they are massaged into the skin.

CHAPTER 2

The Importance of Essential Fatty Acids and Other Nutrients for Beauty and Health

~◞

You see them everywhere: Women lunching on romaine lettuce seasoned with a few drops of lemon juice, men assiduously gnawing skinless, fatless chicken pieces, trying to convince themselves that their "healthy" lunch tastes great. Of all the misconceptions among North Americans today, the no-fat diet trend is truly misguided.

First and foremost, we all need some oil in our diets, for our general health, to promote good looks, and to help make food tasty. The essential fatty acids and essential oils are the incomparable lubricants that make the wheels of life turn more smoothly, strongly, joyfully, and beautifully.

I have no quarrel with low-fat diets; in fact, nearly every doctor, dietitian, and allied health professional agrees that, as a general rule, this is the way to go. But no-fat? This is not only scientifically invalid and actually unhealthy, but signals a self-flagellating, puritanical approach to life that I find disconcerting. And so would most people around the world! Whether it's in my native Jamaica, in the hills of Tuscany, in a rural village in China, or in the mountains of Morocco, food represents much more than sustenance. It is a tie that binds, a communal and daily celebration that pulls people together. Even if we dine alone, it is a time for reflection, celebration, a break from the hectic times in which we live.

Just consider the annals of art and literature, and how full they are of feasts and other celebrations involving food. Rent the divine Danish film *Babette's Feast*, all about the preparation of a feast nonpareil, the wonderful Chinese film *Eat Drink Man Woman*, or the delightful American movie *Big Night*. (And has there ever been a French film on any theme that didn't feature at least one *grand buffet*? I rest my case!) I also have wonderful memories of our family feasts, replete with colors, spices, and heavenly aromas. To this day, I'm mystified by the colorless, tasteless, bland foods that some people eat.

The point is this: When we deny ourselves food in all its richness, we deny ourselves one of the great joys of life. And in the body-obsessed times of today, many people take all pleasure out of eating in the name of good looks, when depriving themselves of wholesome foods may have just the opposite result.

THE ESSENTIAL FATTY ACIDS

Essential is the key word here, and here are the reasons. The health benefits of the essential fatty acids include:

- improved circulation
- lower levels of cholesterol
- ability to cope more easily with stress
- reduction of allergic reactions
- lessened effects of PMS
- stimulation of the immune system
- an aid to longevity

The above are reason enough to incorporate essential fatty acids into your diet. But that's just the start. You can also visibly improve the way you look. Among the wonderful results you'll see are:

- softer, clearer, younger-looking skin
- stronger, faster-growing nails
- shiny, healthy hair
- bright eyes
- better-lubricated muscles and joints

What Are Essential Fatty Acids and
Why Are They Essential?

Essential fatty acids (EFAs) are the basic building blocks of fats in the human body. An important source of energy, fatty acids are the largest structural component of the membrane that surrounds each cell in the human body.

These EFAs not only protect existing cells but also help to build and maintain healthy new cells. For this reason, they are needed from the moment of conception and are important throughout every stage of our development. This is precisely why no-fat diets for pregnant women are extremely dangerous. Moreover, EFAs form the fat surrounding all our internal organs, providing insulation and protection to these organs. Fatty acids are also needed for the creation of important biological regulators called prostaglandins.

Not only are EFAs absolutely essential for optimal health, but they have a huge impact on your physical appearance. Even a mild deficiency of fatty acids can cause your skin to become dry, lined, and leathery, and will make you look far older than you are. Take a look at your friends, colleagues, or associates who are on ultra-low-fat or no-fat diets. See how dull and lifeless their hair looks, no matter how expensive the products they use or how much time they spend at the beauty salon. Consider how blotchy, dry, or dull their skin looks, and how these people often have very fragile nails.

Why is this so? Because EFAs work as internal moisturizing agents, helping you look your best (as well as promoting excellent wellness and health). Others fats may have the opposite effect. Animal fats, especially (with the exception of a little butter), should be minimized or eliminated entirely.

There are two major categories of essential fatty acids: the omega-6 fats and the omega-3 fats.

The Omega-6 Fatty Acids

The omega-6 fats are polyunsaturated fats that are derived from linoleic acid, which is found in almost all vegetable oils, nuts, seeds, and leafy vegetables. If our diets are lacking in linoleic acid, gaps appear within cells, causing loss of moisture and dehydration. If our diets remain deficient in EFAs for long periods of time, even greater health problems can occur: hair loss, eczema, and, at worst, dehydration of various glands, with consequent heart and circulation problems.

Of all the fatty acids, it is linoleic acid, found in both omega-6 and omega-3 fats, that is most required by the human body. It not only keeps our cells functioning at their best but also helps boost our immune systems. A balance between omega-6 and omega-3 fats is important. The typical American diet is far richer in omega-6 oils, and one must make a special effort to include more omega-3 oils. This is most easily done, as the next section suggests, through eating certain fish several times a week.

Omega-3 Fatty Acids:
Health Promoters and Super–Skin Savers

Physicians and anthropologists studying the Eskimos of the Arctic Circle noted that, despite their huge intake of animal fats (chiefly whale blubber, seal meat, and salmon), Eskimos have practically no incidence of heart disease. The researchers discovered that these fatty foods are rich in omega-3 fatty acids, the other essential oil that protects humans from many health problems. In fact, our risk of not only heart disease, but also diabetes and stroke, is greatly reduced when we incorporate omega-3s in our diets. Certain cold-water fish are the richest source of omega-3s, which are also abundant in flaxseed oil.

Fish oils contain two important ingredients, eicosapentaenoic acid (EPA) and docosahexaenoic acid (DHA), which regulate the activity of prostaglandins. These prostaglandins are potent disease fighters that have been shown to keep our bodies healthy.

All of the following fish are rich in omega-3 fatty acids:

- tuna (albacore has a greater concentration of omega-3s than the more inexpensive "light" tuna)
- salmon

- herring

- sardines

- mackerel

At this time, the general consensus is that we should be eating the fish listed above three or four times a week. Chapter 5 features a full range of delicious and healthful recipes that will allow you to reap the full benefits of these wonderful fatty fish oils. Although it is best to eat these fish to enjoy the fullest possible benefits of fish oils, supplements of both fish and flaxseed oil are also available.

Other Benefits of Fish Oils

The good news on essential oils provided by fish just keeps on coming. Among the latest findings:

1. In France, researchers found that fish oil helps relieve the effects of asthma.

2. In England, doctors discovered that the modulation of prostaglandins by omega-3 fatty acids helps control the inflammation of arthritis.

3. Fish oils are also known to reduce the deleterious effects of leukotrienes, which are found in unusually high numbers in people with eczema and psoriasis. Empirical evidence shows that fatty fish oils ease the effects of these debilitating skin ailments.

THE GOOD FATS . . . AND THE BAD ONES

Saturates? Monounsaturates? Polyunsaturates? The good news is that folks all across North America are more enlightened about these fats than ever before. The bad news is that many people are still quite confused. In order to incorporate the "good" essential fatty acids into your daily diet, it is important to understand the differences among them. So take a few minutes to read the next paragraphs carefully.

Saturated Fats

Saturated fats are those fats that are derived from animals and some plant sources. Virtually all saturated fats are solid at room temperature. These saturated fats can block the arteries, causing heart and circulation problems (especially as we age); they also have been found to cause some cancers, especially breast and prostate cancers.

In addition, saturated fats slow down the removal of waste matter and toxins in our bodies by clogging our lymphatic system. This negatively affects the skin by amassing debris, which can lead to pimples, rashes, and a host of other skin ailments, such as bloating, cellulite, and puffiness.

Moreover, North Americans are heavier today than at any other time in history; in fact, as many as 50 percent of Americans are classified as overweight. Not only do many of us eat too much

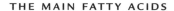

THE MAIN FATTY ACIDS

Saturates	Monounsaturates	Polyunsaturates
lard	olives and olive oil	almonds and almond oil
meat fat and	canola oil	sunflower oil
drippings	peanuts and	safflower oil
whole milk/cream	peanut oil	corn oil
butter	peanut butter	walnuts and walnut oil
cheese	avocado	soybean oil
egg yolk	cashews	fish and fish oil
coconut oil		flaxseed oil
palm oil		
poultry fat		

meat, but many foods we buy are chock-full of these unhealthy saturated fats and heavily laced with salt and refined sugar.

To safeguard your health, animal fats should be eaten only sparingly, and fresh fruits and vegetables eaten raw or lightly steamed should be the mainstay of your diet. Beware, too, of hidden culprits; many saturated fats and harmful chemicals creep into canned, frozen, and other packaged foods. Take a good, hard look at the ingredients list of the products you feed your family before you put them in your shopping cart.

To reduce the amount of saturated fats in your diet:

- Eat more fish and legumes (vegetable protein).
- Reduce your intake of red meat and choose the leanest cuts.
- Remove excess fat when you eat beef, pork, lamb, and veal.

- Replace meat with poultry (chicken, turkey) and remove the fat and skin.
- Grill or roast meats; eliminate frying.
- Use low-fat or skim milk, or soy milk, instead of whole milk or half-and-half.
- Replace mayonnaise with yogurt on sandwiches and when you prepare tuna and chicken salads.
- Increase your usage of herbs and spices (which are wonderful antioxidants and digestive aids) to help undo unhealthy eating habits, while adding pep and taste to your foods.
- Eat more organically grown grains, fresh fruit, and vegetables. These live foods are the "roto-rooter" cleansers of the digestive tract.

Once again, moderation is the key. You needn't be a fanatic. An occasional ice cream indulgence is not a crime. It's better to have one scoop of the real stuff once a month than to eat a whole carton of reduced-fat ice cream three times a week, just as one or two fresh-baked cookies or a French fruit tart every so often is far better than eating a boxful of tasteless SnackWells every other day. You are less likely to see a slim person eating diet cookies or drinking diet soda!

For the same reason, a French person who eats poultry or red meat once a day can afford to eat the skin, especially when her other meal is, typically, vegetable-based, or uses animal protein as just part of a multi-veggie stew. When foreigners come to the United States and see the gargantuan steaks and huge half-chickens considered normal portions here, they look like the Lilliputians did the first time they laid eyes on Gulliver.

Monounsaturated and Polyunsaturated Fats

Both of these types of fats, in moderation, have a place in every healthy diet.

Monounsaturated fats, such as olive oil and others listed in the chart on page 19, are liquid at room temperature but solidify slightly when chilled. Although they are not "essential" in the same way that omega-3s and omega-6s are, they are an important addition to a healthy diet. Research has shown that olive oil in particular may protect against heart disease and cancer.

Polyunsaturated fats, which include vegetable, seed, nut, and fish oils, remain liquid both at room temperature and when refrigerated. Certain polyunsaturated fats are essential for health and wellness, yet these are not manufactured by the human body. Thus, our supply of these oils *must* come from the foods we eat. The amount our bodies require is not large, but it is important that we eat enough of them every single day.

Essential fatty acids help build the fragile membranes surrounding every single human cell. By reinforcing these cell membranes, EFAs also prevent water loss and keep cells healthy and strong. These acids are also required to preserve the protective lipid barrier between the upper and lower levels of our skin, which is precisely why their inclusion in our diets is essential to keeping our skin radiant and young. EFAs encourage the replacement of collagen and elastin in our skin's dermis as well, thus preventing wrinkling and helping to defy gravity's effects.

Be aware that these essential fats are easily destroyed by fat-soluble substances, including alcohol, some prescription (and illicit) drugs, and certain environmental chemicals. Thus, excessive alcohol consumption and recreational drugs should be avoided. Be very cautious also with prescription drugs and environmental chemicals, another good reason to choose organic foods.

WHAT IS WRONG WITH HYDROGENATION?

Hydrogenation combines polyunsaturated fats with hydrogen, which turns them into an unnatural solid state. Most margarines, low-fat yogurt/margarine/butter spreads, and other processed foods are hydrogenated or partially hydrogenated. Thus the chemical structure of once-healthy polyunsaturated oils changes, and they behave like our enemies, the saturated fats, in our bodies.

It is very important that you read food labels carefully. Nearly all mass-distributed margarine products are hydrogenated and should be avoided. Happily, some markets and many health food stores have products that are made with unhydrogenated oils. This is good news, because these products do not alter the basic molecular structure of essential plant oils, thus keeping their health benefits intact.

Other Cautions

Another possible problem with polyunsaturated oils is that their chemical structure breaks down at high temperatures. In this case, peroxides (which damage the body) are the result. For this reason, polyunsaturated oils like sunflower and safflower oil should not be used for frying. Instead, any of the polyunsaturates are excellent used at room temperature (or slightly chilled) in salad dressing and homemade mayonnaise.

On the other hand, monounsaturated oils (such as olive oil, favored by Italians, and sesame oil, beloved by Chinese) are more stable chemically, and thus better for frying or other food preparation requiring heating.

All oils start to spoil via oxidization as soon as the bottles containing them are opened. Therefore, be sure not to leave bottles open longer than necessary and keep them out of the light and away from heat. A dark closet is fine for olive oil, but your refrigerator is better for polyunsaturates.

The best place to buy high-quality cold-pressed oils is in your local health food store, gourmet shop, or the specialty section in your local supermarket. You must read the labels—especially the back label—to know exactly what you are buying.

VITAMIN SUPPLEMENTS

In general, I recommend avoiding mass-distributed, heavily advertised vitamins, because most of these are manufactured from chemically produced synthetic vitamins and minerals. Instead, look for vitamins derived from natural plant sources. I suggest taking a good multivitamin and multimineral every day. Typically, you can find these at health food stores or in health catalogs. Although I do not endorse specific brands, I suggest you cultivate a relationship with knowledgeable salespeople in your local health food store or natural pharmacy. Better yet, consult a nutritionist or a naturopathic physician.

The Importance of Vitamin E

Once upon a time, women and men got all the vitamin E their bodies needed from their diet. Unfortunately, all too often our modern diets are deficient in this essential ingredient for skin health. Overly refined wheat, additives, and preservatives in packaged foods, and chemicals in our soil have taken a terrible toll on the presence of vitamin E in the food we eat.

Of all foodstuffs, wheat germ (or its oil) has the greatest concentration of vitamin E. Why, then, isn't it present in the bread we eat? Because in standard-issue American white bread, the milling and production process depletes up to 90 percent of the wheat's vitamin E content, not to mention the entire B complex of vitamins and several important minerals. Select only whole grain breads and be sure to check the ingredients list.

You can also find vitamin E in cold-pressed vegetable oils. Safflower, corn, and soybean oil are among the very best. But beware: Most supermarket vegetable oils are overly refined, a process that virtually eliminates all the vitamin E. Thus, it is very important to buy cold-pressed unrefined oil; look at the label to make sure. In general, those oils that are darkest are the least refined and thus will have the highest concentration of super-healthful vitamin E.

Oxidation is a chemical reaction that provides the human body's cells with oxygen; as such, it is essential to life itself. But if this process works overtime, it can produce skin damaging free radicals. These volatile particles can come both from within and without. For this very reason, it is essential that we counteract their effects with what we eat and with nutritional supplements, not merely—as the cosmetics behemoths would have it—by slathering cream on our faces. Another way we can slow down the skin's aging processes and provide antioxidant protein to the cells is by using essential oils in our creams, blends, and lotions. See chapter 7.

External and Internal Free Radicals

Internal free radicals are produced by our bodies as oxygen is released. If uncontrolled, they can multiply and actually destroy cells—even DNA, the building block of all human life. What's more, when a free radical attacks a cell, it often combines with polyunsaturated fatty acids. The result of this unfortunate union is lipid peroxides, which generate the production of even more free radicals for a virtual round-robin of cell destruction.

Free radicals are also present in our environment. These include:

- nitrogen dioxide and ozone found in smog and industrial pollution
- lead and other metals
- exhaust fumes from cars, buses, and trucks
- direct sunlight
- cigarette smoke
- pesticides
- food additives and microwave radiation

All these, as you can imagine, are perils of modern life—toxic input began with the Industrial Revolution and has multiplied exponentially in the last century alone. What are the effects of free radicals on our bodies? The negative consequences can include:

- premature aging

- skin (and other) cancers

- cataracts

- dermatitis

- eczema

- immune system suppression

Vitamin E Supplements to the Rescue!

As with any vitamin or nutrient, it is ever so much better to try to derive the benefits of these oils from food you eat. However, given the realities of our modern diet, I believe that it is harder to obtain the required amount of vitamin E than that of any other nutrient or mineral. For this reason, I do recommend a daily vitamin E supplement. The good news is that nearly all well-designed multivitamins exceed the FDA minimum daily requirement of vitamin E. To be sure, check the label of the vitamin you take and make sure that it contains 100 to 400 IU of vitamin E.

CHAPTER 3

Beauty from the Inside Out: The Perfect Beauty Foods

It's become such a cliché, but it's so true: We are what we eat!

Our skin is an almost perfect mirror of our general health. So how can our faces be at their best when we exist on a fast-food diet, or one devoid of fruits, vegetables, and essential fatty acids? The answer is: They usually can't. In fact, it is not only the skin on our faces that suffers when we eat poorly. Most skin conditions, from eczema to psoriasis, are the direct result of imbalances in our bodies, and many are the direct result of poor dietary choices.

That's the bad news. The good news is that the healthy recipes presented here incorporate everything you need to look and feel your very best. Which is precisely why I present the "inside" portion of this book before getting to the "outside" part that presents topical skin preparations and programs.

Better news still is that no matter how old you are, no matter how poorly you have "fed" your face in the past, you can still look fabulous, beginning now. That's because the cells of the skin constantly regenerate themselves, and how you eat today will have a very positive impact on how you look tomorrow.

In the previous chapter, we discussed how important it was to get proper amounts of essential fatty acids and vitamin E from the food that you eat, day in and day out. But there's more to good nutrition than that. There's a whole alphabet of essential vitamins, minerals, amino acids, and phytochemicals that are best gotten from a healthy, balanced diet. Vitamin supplements are helpful, but they can't provide everything your body needs, especially if they are synthetically produced.

An optimally balanced diet should include the following every day:

- five vegetables of different colors, including at least one serving of dark leafy greens
- 1 to 2 tablespoons of uncooked cold-pressed vegetable oil (if fish isn't on the menu, take 1 tablespoon flaxseed oil)
- one to two servings of whole grain bread, grain (brown rice), or cereal
- one small serving of animal or vegetable protein prepared with herbs and spices at every meal

- two to three different fresh fruits
- six to eight glasses of plain (not carbonated) water

FOODS TO AVOID

Sugar

Excess refined sugars should be avoided at all times. There have been so many articles and books written about the dangers of consuming an overload of refined sugar that I hesitate to join the clamor. However, a swift recap of the commonsense reasons for such avoidance includes:

- energy fluctuations
- tooth decay
- overweight

- blood sugar problems
- skin eruptions

Processed Juices

Limit your intake of processed juices. One of the most common American misconceptions is that it is healthy to drink orange juice every morning and to fill your children with other processed juices from concentrates all day long. Most supermarket juices are concentrates made from large quantities of fruit, many of which are quite acidic. These commercially prepared juices also have the disadvantage of having been homogenized and stabilized (some of them are actually boiled); this leads to even more acidity in the juice and in our systems. It is not unusual to get an almost instant stomachache after chugging down some "healthy" cartoned orange juice. In fact, many people who think they suffer from food allergies to oranges are in fact only allergic to its manufactured juice.

Acidic fruits such as oranges and grapefruits should be eaten in their natural state. It is far better to eat one fresh orange or the freshly prepared juice of one, if the craving for citrus strikes you. That way, you get the benefit of the juice, the orange's fiber, and the whole feeling of the fruit, with nary a twinge in your stomach.

The above said, it is also true that juicing fresh fruits and vegetables can be a healthy addition to the diet. But overindulgence in processed juices leads to burping, gas, and bloating, not to mention a sugar overload, bowel problems, and skin eruptions. If everyone substituted a glass or bottle of water for the endless sodas and fruit juices consumed, the United States would be a far healthier place!

Milk and Dairy Products

Another major misconception is that it is quite all right to eat large quantities of cheese and to drink as much milk as you like. Frankly, many health professionals agree that milk is for growing calves, not humans, although I must admit that it can be quite delicious (as an occasional treat) in some of its prepared forms: yogurt, cream, ice cream, smoothies. Cheese (even the unprocessed varieties), just like juices, milk, and nuts, is a concentrated food that can also lead to clogging and acidosis when eaten to excess.

"But what about calcium?" everyone asks. First of all, the calcium in milk is not well absorbed. Second, you can get adequate amounts of calcium from broccoli and other dark leafy greens, almonds, sardines, and most whole plant foods, not to mention a good supplement. Also, calcium can be absorbed from the essential oils you apply daily to your body (see chapter 6).

Fast Foods

Don't even get me started on the fast foods that pass for lunch and dinner in this country (and, dishearteningly, at an increasing rate in other parts of the world as well). If you cut out just one fast-food meal a day and substituted a healthy home-cooked one, you would very quickly and easily begin your steady journey toward good health and better looks. Chapter 5 offers a marvelous range of recipes and food plans that are quick and easy, yet delicious and beautiful to the eye. I want nature's best food, in all its tasty bounty, to become commonplace for you, as it was for me while I was growing up in Jamaica.

FOODS TO ENJOY

Let's look at the foods you *should* be eating for optimal health and beauty. These are my favorites—those that I eat myself and that I advise my clients to eat. You'll note that vegetables come first, as well they should. I have long believed that fruits and vegetables should provide at least half of any meal, with protein and carbohydrates/grains each contributing another fourth.

My top food choices for good health are:

- green, leafy vegetables (romaine lettuce, kale, spinach, watercress)
- orange-colored vegetables (carrots, pumpkin, yams, squash)
- red-colored vegetables (red bell peppers, beets, tomatoes)
- other green vegetables (broccoli, string beans, green squash, cucumbers, cabbage, bok choy)
- yellow vegetables (corn, yellow squash, yellow peppers)
- beans (kidney, garbanzo, black, lentils, split peas, soybeans)
- whole grains (breads, pasta, brown rice, bulgur wheat, oats, basmati rice)
- proteins (chicken, fish, tofu, nuts, eggs, and dairy eaten sparingly)
- fruits (apples, bananas, pears, mangoes, oranges, papayas, plums, peaches)
- six to eight 8-ounce glasses of water daily

- healthy fats (olive oil, avocados, flaxseed oil, sesame oil)
- herbs and spices (garlic, onions, scallions, thyme, basil, bay, cayenne, dill, cinnamon, nutmeg)
- various sprouts, seeds, and mushrooms
- beverages including water, herb teas, a little coffee if you wish (one cup a day will not kill you), grape juice from time to time (if you must have juice, make it yourself at home)
- small occasional helpings of "devilish" foods that satisfy your soul

Most of all, never fail to carry with you an appreciative attitude toward the foods that are sustaining you and keeping you healthy.

How Can I Add Vital Plant Oils to My Diet?

Salad dressings are the easiest way to make sure you're getting your daily 2 tablespoons of essential fatty acids. There are several wonderful recipes in chapter 5.

Remember that any oil you buy should be either "cold-pressed" or "unprocessed." If you do not find these words on the label, do not put the product in your shopping cart! With this important proviso in mind, here's what you should know about vegetable, seed, and nut oils.

Corn Oil

The least expensive cooking oil on the market, corn oil can be a good source of polyunsaturated fatty acids. However, much of the supermarket corn oil is heavily refined. Look for the unrefined cold-pressed variety available in most health food stores or upscale grocery emporia.

Unrefined corn oil contains a high amount of vitamin E and is an excellent source of linoleic acid and other omega-6 acids. But do beware: Because all polyunsaturated oils break down at high temperatures and release free radical peroxides, it is recommended that you only use corn oil cold (smoothies are the best way, I think). Keep it refrigerated and never use it for cooking.

Olive Oil

How can I add to the harmony of voices praising olive oil? Used for centuries in the Mediterranean, this wonderful oil has only recently started gaining widespread acceptance in this country. Olive oil's sophisticated, light flavoring makes it a perfect candidate for salad dressings and sauces. Moreover, since this is a monounsaturated oil, it can also be used for recipes that require heating—either sautéing or frying.

Several varieties of olive oil are available. Extra virgin olive oil, the best kind, is taken from the first pressing of the olives and contains the most distinctive olive taste. Although a couple of tablespoons for sautéing (often supplemented with butter) won't break the bank, extra virgin olive oil is too expensive to use for frying when a large amount is required. This is a job best left to virgin olive oil, the next-best category. Its color and taste are lighter than extra virgin, but it is just as rich in essential olive oil and nutrients.

By the way, olive oil is one of the only kinds of oil that you can keep in a pantry or cupboard without its becoming rancid. However, it is always best to keep any oil away from direct sunlight. The extremely strong smell and taste can be a turnoff for some people; you can always mix it with another, lighter monounsaturated oil like canola oil.

Safflower Oil

One of the least expensive of all cooking oils, safflower oil is high in polyunsaturates and omega-6 fatty acids. (Caution: As a polyunsaturate, safflower oil should not be used for cooking.) It also contains high amounts of vitamin E. Safflower oil is noted for its deep, nutty taste; as such, it is perfect for salad dressings and sauces. Once again, look for the unrefined variety you'll find in most health food stores. Keep it refrigerated.

Sesame Oil

Sesame seeds are a great natural source of calcium and iron, properties that remain in the oil form. The Chinese, especially, have known about the health benefits of sesame for centuries. Because sesame oil is monounsaturated, it can be used for sautéing without the formation of free radicals. Unrefined sesame oil is the best kind and should always be kept in the refrigerator.

Hazelnut Oil

This is a trendy new addition to American cupboards and a welcome one. The best hazelnut oil comes from Provence, where it is lovingly pressed and filtered by hand. Because it is monounsaturated, hazelnut is a good, though expensive, cooking oil.

Sunflower Oil

The oil extracted from sunflower seeds is light and sweet. Unrefined sunflower oil contains high levels of linoleic acid and omega-6 essential fatty acids, as well as moderate amounts of vitamin E. It is polyunsaturated, and thus best used cold in dressings. Sunflower oil should always be refrigerated to prevent spoilage.

Walnut Oil

This traditional favorite among French chefs has only recently been introduced to North America. It is expensive, but its nutty flavor goes a long way. It is a wonderful addition to omelets and other egg dishes; many cooks use it to flavor desserts. Always keep unrefined walnut oil in your refrigerator.

THE MAGIC OF CULINARY HERBS

As a former vegetarian and one who still believes in the virtue of an almost meat-free diet, I must say that, until recently, I felt that most vegetarian recipes were fairly tasteless, because they usually were not prepared with spices and herbs. Among some vegetarians, there is a mistaken belief that adding spices to vegetarian foods can somehow pollute their purity. Nothing could be further from the truth. In fact, herbs (found naturally in temperate regions) and spices (found naturally in tropical and subtropical regions) have the important jobs of:

- exciting the palate and sense of smell
- destroying microbes and parasites in foods
- aiding efficient digestion of foods
- adding important vitamins and antioxidants to the diet

- cleaning and toning the liver, gallbladder, and spleen
- speeding up the removal of waste products by the colon

Try adding a dash of cinnamon, nutmeg, or allspice to mashed potatoes, a baked squash, or yam, and see how delicious it is!

WHAT ABOUT MEAT?

I include chicken and fish in my weekly food plan, although vegetables, fruits, and grains should be the backbone of a healthy diet. Follow the guidelines cited earlier. After years of research and personal eating experience, I believe that this is the optimal way to nourish yourself both inside and out.

Although red meat is not for me, I do believe you can eat it once or twice a week in small servings without any ill effects. But no more than that; almost all the livestock we eventually eat are force-fed antibiotics, steroids, pesticide-laden grains, and who knows what else. If you do plan to eat red meat, I suggest the following guidelines:

- Only buy organic meat.
- Assiduously avoid organ meats (brains, liver, kidney, sweetbreads), which are home to all kinds of toxins. This is especially true of the liver, which acts as a detoxifier, and the kidney, which filters impurities from the system.

- Lean cuts of meat are always best.

- Remove all excess fat before cooking.

- Broiling or grilling meat is not as healthy as commonly thought; instead, roast your meats at low temperatures (350 degrees Fahrenheit is best) and always use a drip pan to catch excess grease.

Moderation is, as always, the key. And that, friends, is my view on the vegetarian issue!

CHAPTER 4

CLEANSING FASTS AND RECIPES

~⌒

I CAN STILL REMEMBER READING MY SISTER'S MOVIE MAGAZINES AS A young girl. Thinking back, it's clear to see why I became an aromatherapist: It wasn't the stories of fame or fortune that interested me, but the eccentric yet fascinating health and beauty tips given by the movie stars of the day. There seemed to be no end to the fasts, salts, and diets they followed to look gorgeous and stay young forever!

Of course, as I continued my studies of aromatherapy, cell biology, and natural healing, I learned more and more about holistic wellness programs that had seemed so glamorous while growing up. Then, starting in the '70s—with a brief nod to the '60s!—the health revolution began in earnest. I began to see a welcome fusion of healthy eating within the now-named holistic health movement. It was interesting, too, to see the evolution of how alternative health practices were reported by the general press: What started as derision ended with reverence, and today more than 40 percent of Americans report they have tried at least one alternative health therapy in the past year. Alternative health is on the cover of major news magazines, and books like those by Dr. Andrew Weil have topped all the best-seller lists.

All this is a necessary preamble to this chapter. Like many alternative therapies, the subject of cleansing regimens might have been greeted with circumspection just a few decades ago. Not so today, when even the most conventional of doctors is beginning to recommend these programs as part of a patient's general wellness program.

Fasts and cleansing regimens are an especially important way of clearing our systems as we undertake any new health lifestyle—and your new way of looking at beauty certainly constitutes that! So let's look at my favorite ways to help normalize the body, the perfect preparation to a lifetime of essential beauty.

WHY FAST?

The first and most important reason to fast is to give your system a rest. An enormous amount of energy goes into digesting foods, especially the protein- and fat-rich fast-food diets of so many Americans. Thus, energy is taken away from other parts of the body in order to accomplish what should be the natural act of digestion.

Second, any digested food can become poisonous if it stays in the colon for too long. The fiber-deficient fast foods many people eat are among the main culprits here. These so-called foods stay in the colon for much, much longer than they should. Fruits and vegetables are the "roto-rooters" of the colon; these natural wonders get waste products moving and out of the body.

When we are not eliminating toxins quickly enough, we tend to feel bloated, constipated, sluggish, dull, and, in the worst case scenario, downright ill. This is because virtually all our energy seems to be at work in our tummy, lower back, and legs. The unhappy result is that we feel irritable and can lose mental focus, and our sinuses and lungs can seem clogged. The latter happens because of the mucous blockage that emanates from the digestive tract.

At the same time, the skin can look dull, thickened, and discolored, because it is not getting enough vital nutrients from the liver (which itself is struggling to cope with toxic overloads). As a result, the skin, too, is unable do one of its most important jobs, that of eliminating toxins through the pores. So, our skin becomes depleted or even sick.

To rectify these problems, a healthy lifestyle changeover, begun and/or maintained by periodic juice fasting, is one of the best things we can do for our bodies—and for our looks. A successful fast leads to improved circulation, uplifted energy, healthier skin, and clearer eyes.

If you have been overindulging in processed foods and are constipated, you should take an herbal laxative before starting the fast. This is important because without the bulk of food passing through the colon before fasting, the muscles can relax too much and not contract sufficiently to get waste products out of the body.

A Good Cleansing Hint

Before you begin your day, put a slice of lemon or lime in a cup of hot water and drink it. This is a wonderful way of eliminating stale digestive juices and gases from the digestive track and helps cleanse the liver as well. My mother had my whole family do this, and I firmly believe that we are all healthier for doing so.

JUICE FASTS

First, let's start with some wonderful juice fasts that will clear out and regulate your system and help get your body back in fighting shape.

Before we begin, several words of caution:

- Diabetics should avoid these programs because fruits contain fructose, which is a form of sugar.

- If you have an extremely acid system or suffer from arthritis, cellulite, or kidney stones, avoid orange and grapefruit juices. Even though lemons and limes are also citrus, they become alkaline when they enter the digestive tract; hence, my suggestion to drink hot water with lemon first thing in the morning.

- People suffering from chronic or acute health problems should consult their physicians before undertaking a fast or cleansing regimen of any kind.

For most of us, happily, juice fasts are in no way detrimental to our general health. Indeed, quite the opposite is true. Fasts can improve our general state of well-being and the way we feel. The wonderful thing about completing a one- or two-day juice fast is that you feel so clean and virtuous. But to fully reap the benefits of these fasts, you must start with a clean colon. Otherwise, constipation is likely to occur, because there is just not enough peristaltic movement in digesting juices. Thus, I suggest drinking an herbal tea like cascara sagrada or taking herbal laxative tablets the night before you start your juice fast.

When to do a fast? Whenever your overall health is good, but you feel stressed, clogged, tired, or overanxious, or in any other way need to jump-start your system.

To make these juices, you need a heavy-duty automatic juicer, one that leaves very little pulp behind.

✄ VEGETABLE JUICE FAST

1 cup water
2 carrots
1 stick celery
1 handful parsley
1 beet
1 teaspoon flaxseed oil
½ teaspoon grated fresh ginger

In a blender or juicer, blend together all ingredients except ginger at medium speed until smooth. Add the ginger and blend for a few seconds longer. Drink one glass immediately at room temperature; save the other, covered, in the refrigerator for later.

✄ FRUIT JUICE FAST

1 Bosc or other pear, cored and chopped
3 apricots or peaches, pitted and chopped
1 banana, chopped
½ organic lemon with peel, chopped
1 plum, pitted and chopped
½ cup water
½ teaspoon nutmeg or cinnamon

Mix all ingredients in a blender at medium speed until smooth. Drink immediately, at room temperature.

ORANGE-MANGO FAST TREAT

- 1 orange, peeled, seeded, and sectioned
- 1 tangerine, peeled, seeded, and sectioned
- 5 or 6 strawberries or pitted cherries
- 1 handful grapes
- 1 ripe mango, pitted and diced
- ½ cup water
- ¼ teaspoon cinnamon

Blend all ingredients together at medium speed until smooth. Drink immediately.

COMBO VEGGIE/JUICE FAST

- ½ cup water
- 2 carrots
- 1 beet
- 3 leaves spinach
- 1 banana
- ½ lemon
- 1 teaspoon olive oil
- ¼ teaspoon vanilla

Blend together at medium speed until smooth. Drink immediately.

How Much Juice to Drink

During your first fast day, you can drink up to four 8-ounce glasses of juice, diluted with water if you wish. Also, drink plenty of water and herbal teas during the day. If you wish, for variety's sake you can substitute hot, unsalted, clear vegetable broth for one of the juice drinks.

It is possible that you will feel extremely hungry on the first day of this fast. Unless you are a diabetic, hypoglycemic, or under a doctor's care, try to work through this feeling. It is not going to kill you to do without food for a limited amount of time, and you will do your digestive organs, circulation, and skin a world of good by undertaking this fast. To quell your hunger, I suggest sipping hot herb tea with nutmeg, ginger, or cinnamon as often as you like.

FRUIT FASTS

If a juice fast seems too difficult for you now, try these two fruit-only fasts that are effective colon cleansers as well.

Grape and Apple System Cleanser

For two days, alternate purple grapes and red apples as your food source. Supplement with at least eight 8-ounce glasses of lemon water per day and hot herbal teas or unsalted vegetable broths.

Plum 'n' Prune One-Day Fast

Though this works far better if you stay on this fast for two days, one day is better than none. At any rate, it provides a good introduction to the glories of fasting. Alternately eat plums, prunes, and prune juice (with a dash of cinnamon) and drink only pure spring water (again, eight 8-ounce glasses are recommended). This is quite a delicious fast and one that I heartily recommend.

CHAPTER 5

SKIN-SATIONAL RECIPES

THE PROBLEM WITH MOST FOOD PLANS PRESENTED IN HEALTH AND beauty books is that they're too boring for words. Either that, or the recipes are too complicated for anyone other than Julia Child or Emeril Lagasse! For that reason, I've kept the choices here so simple that even a kitchen novice could prepare them with ease. The recipes that follow are immensely savory and flavorful and represent the best-loved cuisines from everywhere on Earth, including my native Jamaica. Since we don't have time in our busy schedules to prepare a full-blown lunch, I sometimes suggest healthy choices of foods you can easily buy at grocery stores, delis, and coffee shops wherever you live.

It is very important to eat two to three pieces of fresh fruit during the day. In some of the menu plans, I mention fruit smoothies as a way of ensuring fruit variety, but you should make a conscious effort to eat two to three different kinds of fruit daily as snacks or desserts.

DAILY MENUS

Recipes for those dishes marked with an asterisk (*) follow.

DAY 1

BREAKFAST: *Breakfast Smoothie and 2 slices whole wheat toast

LUNCH: Turkey and bean burrito with mixed green salad and German potato salad

DINNER: *Japanese Salmon Steak with steamed vegetable medley and brown rice

DAY 2

BREAKFAST: Hot oatmeal with raisins and cinnamon

LUNCH: *Creamy Broccoli Soup with whole wheat crackers

DINNER: *Lazy Man's Roast Chicken with brussels sprouts, steamed carrots, and mixed salad

DAY 3

BREAKFAST: Melon balls with raisins, soft-boiled egg, whole wheat toast, and organic coffee

LUNCH: *Provençal Chicken Salad with Mustard Vinaigrette Dressing

DINNER: *Hawaiian-Style Baked Fish with *Gingered Carrots and steamed broccoli

DAY 4

BREAKFAST: Apple juice with cinnamon, banana, corn muffin, and green or black tea

LUNCH: Turkey burger (no bun) with four whole-grain crackers, garden salad with *Herbed Dressing, and one scoop fruit sorbet

DINNER: *Pasta with Fresh Tomato Sauce, crusty Italian bread

DAY 5

BREAKFAST: Whole wheat French toast with cinnamon and maple syrup, apple, organic coffee

LUNCH: Chicken vegetable soup with whole wheat roll, shredded carrot, and raisin salad

DINNER: *Lili's Oriental Baked Chicken, rice, and steamed broccoli and yellow squash

DAY 6

BREAKFAST: Fresh orange, quartered; 1 cup cooked oatmeal with cinnamon and raisins; peppermint tea

LUNCH: Tuna in vegetable oil (3-ounce can), hard-boiled egg, mixed salad, one slice whole wheat bread, and ½ cup strawberry yogurt

DINNER: *Jamaican Escovetched Fish with cornbread, steamed vegetables, steamed plantains, and salad

DAY 7

BREAKFAST: *Algerian-Style Eggs

LUNCH: *Crabmeat Salad Vinaigrette with all-grain roll

DINNER: *Country-Style Chicken Kiev with baked potatoes, yellow squash, *Green Garden Salad with *Herbed Flaxseed Oil Dressing, and *Strawberry Sorbet

RECIPES

DAY 1

❧ BREAKFAST SMOOTHIE

 1 banana
 1 handful ripe berries
 3 tablespoons plain yogurt
 1 tablespoon Missing Link powder*
 ¼ cup water or soy milk
 3 drops ginseng extract
 1 tablespoon olive or flax oil
 ¼ lemon

Place all ingredients in blender. Mix at high speed for 3 minutes, or until smooth. Serve immediately. You may keep unused portions in the refrigerator for later use. Serve with 2 slices whole wheat toast with a small pat of sweet organic butter for energy and stamina to spare!

Yield: 1 serving

*Missing Link powder is among my favorite finds. It is a creation of Dr. Udo Erasmus and contains all the essential vitamins, minerals, and trace elements our bodies need daily.

DAY 1

✄ JAPANESE SALMON STEAK

2 tablespoons teriyaki sauce

¼ cup white wine or vermouth

1 clove garlic, crushed

1 salmon steak, approximately 6 ounces

2 teaspoons olive oil

Preheat oven to 350 degrees F. To prepare the sauce, mix teriyaki sauce, white wine or vermouth, and crushed garlic in a small bowl. Marinate salmon in the sauce for at least 1 hour; better still, marinate in your refrigerator overnight.

Lay salmon steak on top of the olive oil in an oven-proof dish. Bake at 350 degrees, turning once, for 15 minutes or until done. Serve immediately with a steamed medley of broccoli, onion, carrots, and peas, accompanied by ½ cup cooked brown rice.

Yield: 1 serving

DAY 2

✂ CREAMY BROCCOLI SOUP

10	ounces frozen chopped broccoli or 2 cups fresh florets
2	garlic cloves, halved
1	medium onion, chopped
15	ounces chicken broth
2	tablespoons lemon juice
1	cup plain yogurt
½	cup soy milk
½	teaspoon powdered nutmeg
	Salt and pepper to taste

Place broccoli, garlic, onion, and 2 tablespoons chicken broth in a microwavable dish. Microwave, covered, on high until onions are soft (10 to 12 minutes), stopping once to break up frozen broccoli (if used). Or, cook above items on stove top in covered saucepan over medium heat, adding 1 tablespoon water, for 15 minutes.

Put cooked vegetables, lemon juice, and remaining broth in blender; puree. Blend in yogurt, soy milk, and seasonings. Chill and serve with croutons or whole wheat crackers.

Yield: 4 servings

DAY 2

✄ LAZY MAN'S ROAST CHICKEN

1 whole chicken, approximately 3 pounds
Poultry seasoning
Black pepper

Preheat oven to 350 degrees F. Take the bag of innards out of the chicken. Wash chicken thoroughly. Sprinkle liberally with poultry seasoning, available in any grocery. Sprinkle with more black pepper if you like your food spicy.

Place chicken, wing side up, on roasting pan. After half an hour, baste with juices; do so every 15 minutes until done. Check chicken after 1 hour; if juices run clear, it is done. If you like chicken more well done, leave in 10 minutes longer. Serve with brussels sprouts seasoned with a bit of butter, salt, and pepper; steamed carrots; and mixed salad.

Yield: 2 to 4 servings

DAY 3

✂ PROVENÇAL CHICKEN SALAD
WITH MUSTARD VINAIGRETTE DRESSING

This recipe comes from Mike Ahern, a psychologist by vocation and a master chef by avocation.

        2   tablespoons red wine vinegar
        1   tablespoon Dijon mustard
        6   tablespoons olive oil
        ⅛   teaspoon salt
            Pepper to taste
        2   tablespoons fresh tarragon, chopped
        1   head each Boston and red leaf lettuce
12 to 18   ounces shredded chicken meat (light and dark)
            Steamed green beans, sliced red pepper strips,
              and sliced ripe tomatoes

To prepare dressing, combine the first six ingredients in a bowl and whisk together. In a separate large bowl, toss the lettuce in enough of the dressing to lightly coat all leaves. Arrange the dressed lettuce on a platter large enough to accommodate it Top decoratively with the shredded chicken and vegetables. Sprinkle with additional chopped fresh herbs, if desired. Serve immediately.

Yield: 4 to 6 servings

DAY 3

✂ HAWAIIAN-STYLE BAKED FISH

2   pounds fresh or frozen fish fillets, thawed,
     such as cod or halibut
3   tablespoons butter
3   tablespoons flour
2   cups soy milk
1   8-ounce can crushed pineapple
    Salt and pepper to taste
1   teaspoon curry powder
¼   teaspoon ground ginger
¼   cup shredded coconut
3   cups cooked rice

Place fish fillets in a shallow baking pan. In a separate pot, melt butter and stir in flour. Whisk in soy milk and all other ingredients except rice. Bring to a boil and simmer 5 minutes. Pour this mixture over fish and bake 15 minutes at 350 degrees F. Serve fish and sauce on top of cooked rice.

Yield: 6 servings

DAY 3

GINGERED CARROTS

1½ pounds carrots, diced
1   tablespoon sesame or hazelnut oil
5   tablespoons water or vegetable stock
¼   teaspoon grated fresh gingerroot
½   teaspoon arrowroot, mixed with 3 tablespoons water
    Salt and pepper to taste
    Chopped fresh parsley as garnish

Sauté the carrots in the oil. Add the water or stock and grated ginger, cover, and simmer until tender. Stir in the diluted arrowroot and simmer for another 1 or 2 minutes, or until smooth and creamy. Season with salt and pepper, sprinkle with chopped parsley, and serve immediately.

Yield: 4 servings

DAY 4

✄ HERBED DRESSING

    2   tablespoons olive oil
    1   teaspoon plum or fruit vinegar
    1   teaspoon water
    ½   teaspoon mustard or ketchup
    1   dash each powdered ginger, garlic, oregano, black pepper

Mix all ingredients in a small bowl, then pour over freshly prepared salad greens, boiled potatoes, or other vegetables.

Dressing Variations

- Flaxseed oil is a marvelous addition to smoothies and shakes. You'll never know it's there.
- 1 tablespoon of sesame, walnut, almond, or flaxseed oil enhances yogurt or cottage cheese. You can also add these oils to crème fraîche and serve over fresh berries as a dessert!
- Stir 1 teaspoon of hazelnut or almond oil into plain or vanilla yogurt for a delicious treat.
- Add your choice of oil to steamed vegetables. Or stir-fry veggies in 1 tablespoon sesame oil over a high flame for 2 minutes, then cover and steam for 3 or 4 minutes more.

DAY 4

✴ PASTA WITH FRESH TOMATO SAUCE

- 8   ripe, large, off-the-vine tomatoes
- 2   tablespoons olive oil
- ½   medium onion, chopped
- 1   tablespoon garlic, minced
- 1   pound spaghetti (brands imported from Italy are best)
- 1   cup fresh basil, rolled and cut in ⅛-inch strips
      (cut at the last minute to avoid discoloration)
- ¼   cup grated Parmesan cheese
      Salt and pepper to taste

To prepare sauce, immerse the tomatoes in boiling water for 8 seconds. Remove, and when cool enough to handle, slip the skins off. Cut the skinned tomatoes in quarters and gently squeeze the juice and seeds out. Coarsely chop the peeled and seeded tomatoes.

Heat the oil in a large skillet over low heat until hot but not smoking. Add the chopped onion, stirring occasionally until golden. Add the garlic and heat until the garlic takes on a yellow-golden color. Immediately add the tomatoes and turn gently and constantly until they are warmed but not cooked. (If they are allowed to cook, the tomatoes will release their moisture, and the sauce will not succeed.) Remove from heat and put the sauce in a large, warm bowl.

While making the sauce, boil 6 quarts of water with 2 tablespoons salt. Immerse the spaghetti in the water, return to a boil, and let cook until the pasta is cooked al dente—still firm to the tooth when tested. Drain and toss the pasta with the tomato sauce and the shredded basil. Serve with grated Parmesan cheese on the side.

Yield: 4 servings

DAY 5

✂ LILI'S ORIENTAL BAKED CHICKEN

- ½ lemon
- 1 whole 3-pound chicken, cleaned
- ½ teaspoon powdered ginger
- ½ teaspoon black pepper
- 1 teaspoon powdered onion
- ½ cup soy sauce
- 2 tablespoons olive oil

Squeeze lemon all over chicken and rub on outside and inside cavity. Mix ginger, black pepper, and powdered onion. Rub mixture outside skin and inside cavity of chicken. Pour ¼ cup soy sauce into cavity of chicken. Pour remaining soy sauce all over outside of bird.

Pour 1 tablespoon olive oil in baking pan. Place chicken on top. Pour remaining oil over chicken. Bake in preheated oven at 350 degrees F for 1¼ hours, basting frequently. When outside of chicken is golden brown and juice runs clear, it is done. Serve with rice and steamed broccoli and yellow squash.

Yield: 3 to 4 servings

DAY 6

✁ JAMAICAN ESCOVETCHED FISH

6	porgies or 2 small snappers, sliced
1	teaspoon salt
1	teaspoon black pepper
3	tablespoons olive oil
1	large onion, sliced
¼	cup whole peppercorns
1	chili pepper, sliced
¼	cup wine vinegar

Wash fish and pat dry. Season with salt and pepper. Heat heavy saucepan. Add olive oil. Heat to smoking; add fish. Cook on one side for approximately 5 minutes, then flip over and cook for 5 minutes more. Remove fish from heat. Place on a platter. Fry onion in remaining oil (about 5 minutes or until golden). Add peppercorns and sliced chili pepper; remove from fire. Add vinegar, stirring for a few minutes. Pour the marinade over fish. Let sit for a few hours before serving. Serve with cornbread, steamed vegetables, steamed plantains,* and salad.

Yield: 4 to 6 servings

*Plantain (platano) is a tropical vegetable that looks like a large banana. It is never eaten raw because it is indigestible; most commonly in the Caribbean, it is fried. Plantain is also extremely delicious steamed in its skin for approximately 10 minutes (and of course, this is far healthier than frying). If bought with yellow skins, plantains should be put in a paper bag until the skin turns black. This should take 1 to 3 days. Only then should they be cooked; the flavor has developed by this time, and the carotene in the pulp is now ready for the body to absorb.

DAY 7

✖ ALGERIAN-STYLE EGGS

1½ cups canned tomatoes, drained

2 garlic cloves, crushed

1 green pepper, sliced

1 tablespoon butter

6 eggs

½ tablespoon salt

Pepper to taste

Sauté tomatoes with garlic for 5 minutes. Put in buttered 8-inch pie pan. Cook green pepper in butter for 5 minutes or until tender. Put on top of tomatoes. Beat eggs with salt and pepper until well mixed. Pour over tomatoes. Bake in preheated oven at 350 degrees F for 25 minutes or until set.

Yield: 4 servings

DAY 7

✄ CRABMEAT SALAD VINAIGRETTE

    Romaine lettuce
1 6-ounce can crabmeat (or fresh, if possible)
    Diced red peppers and carrots
1 hard-boiled egg, chopped
1 small onion, sliced
    Newman's Own Balsamic Vinaigrette

This is a great take-to-work lunch—delicious, yet easy. Simply wash and tear apart the lettuce, then add crabmeat, peppers, carrots, egg, and onion. Toss with dressing.

Yield: 1 serving

DAY 7

✖ COUNTRY-STYLE CHICKEN KIEV

- ¼ cup sesame oil
- ½ cup fine dry bread crumbs
- 2 teaspoons grated Parmesan cheese
- 1 teaspoon basil
- 1 teaspoon oregano
- ½ teaspoon garlic powder
- ¼ teaspoon cayenne
- ½ teaspoon salt
- 2 chicken breasts, split
- ¼ cup dry white wine
- ¼ cup scallions, chopped
- 1¼ cup parsley, chopped
- 1 tablespoon butter, melted

Preheat oven to 375 degrees F. Put oil on plate.

Combine bread crumbs, Parmesan cheese, basil, oregano, garlic, cayenne, and salt on a piece of wax paper. Dip chicken breasts in oil, then roll in crumbs to coat.

Place chicken skin side up in 9-inch square baking dish. Bake near center of oven for 50 to 60 minutes, or until golden brown and tender.

Meanwhile, add wine, scallions, and parsley to melted butter. When chicken is golden brown, pour butter sauce mixture around and over chicken. Return to oven for 5 minutes longer, or just until sauce is hot. Spoon additional sauce over chicken and serve.

Yield: 4 servings

DAY 7

✄ GREEN GARDEN SALAD

½ cup frozen or fresh green peas
1 small head romaine lettuce
½ small head Boston lettuce
1 small head radicchio lettuce
1 scallion, chopped
1 small cucumber, thinly sliced
1 celery stalk, thinly sliced
½ small bunch watercress

Gently steam peas for 3 minutes. Drain and cool. In a large bowl, tear lettuce into bite-size pieces; add peas, scallion, cucumber, celery, and watercress. Toss salad with Herbed Flaxseed Oil Dressing to coat.

✄ HERBED FLAXSEED OIL DRESSING

¼ cup flaxseed oil
3 tablespoons wine vinegar
1 tablespoon maple syrup
1 tablespoon chopped parsley
½ teaspoon garlic powder
¼ teaspoon powdered oregano
1 teaspoon soy sauce

Shake all ingredients together in a small lidded jar.

Yield: 6 servings

DAY 7

✄ CAULIFLOWER CURRY

1 tablespoon sesame oil

1 large onion, chopped

2 garlic cloves, chopped

½ teaspoon ground turmeric

½ teaspoon ground cumin

1 teaspoon ground coriander seeds

1 fresh green chili pepper, seeds removed, chopped

½ cup cashew nuts

1 cauliflower, divided into florets

¼ cup water

Heat the oil gently in a saucepan. Sauté the onion and garlic for 5 minutes or until translucent. Stir in the turmeric, cumin, coriander, chili pepper, and cashews, and cook for 1 more minute, then add the cauliflower and water. Cover and simmer for 20 minutes, checking during cooking to see that the liquid does not boil away completely (add more water if required).

Yield: 4 servings

DESSERTS

I am the last person in the world to deprive myself of dessert when I really have a hankering for something sweet. In fact, desserts can actually be healthful, especially when they make use of vital plant oils. After all, it's not the sweetness per se that makes many typical American desserts so unhealthy; rather, it's the massive amounts of sugar, artificial flavors, and—in the case of store-bought confections and cakes—preservatives and hydrogenated oils.

Here are my favorite desserts.

✖ ORANGES SUZETTE

4 oranges, peeled and sliced into rounds
½ cup orange juice
1 tablespoon sugar
2 tablespoons Grand Marnier
1 tablespoon brandy

Place orange slices, juice, and sugar in skillet; cook about 2 minutes over medium heat. Stir in Grand Marnier, then add brandy and ignite with a long match. Remove from heat and place orange slices on warmed dessert plates. Spoon additional sauce over fruit and serve. Vanilla yogurt makes the perfect accompaniment to this delightful dessert.

Yield: 4 servings

✄ PEARS HELEN

3 ripe medium pears, peeled, cored, and halved
½ cup hot water
3 tablespoons brown sugar
1 teaspoon butter
3 tablespoons cocoa
2 tablespoons water
3 tablespoons sugar
1 tablespoon Kahlua liqueur
½ cup half-and-half
1 quart vanilla ice milk
1 tablespoon ground almonds
8 ounces sesame seeds
4 ounces rolled oats

Place pears in steamer inside large pot. Combine ½ cup hot water, brown sugar, and butter; pour over fruit. Cover and bring to a boil. Reduce heat and simmer for 20 minutes or until pears are soft. Cool pears in uncovered pot.

Chocolate sauce: In a separate pan, combine cocoa and 2 tablespoons water. Stir to form a smooth paste. Stir in sugar and Kahlua and bring just to a boil. Immediately reduce heat; simmer 5 minutes. Add half-and-half; simmer for 10 minutes more.

To serve, divide ice milk among six dessert plates. Drain pears and place one each on top, round side up. Pour chocolate sauce over pears and sprinkle with almonds, sesame seeds, and rolled oats.

Yield: 6 servings

✂ FRESH FRUIT PARFAIT

1   quart soy milk
½   cup pure maple syrup
6   tablespoons agar flakes
¼   teaspoon sea salt
1   teaspoon vanilla
¼   teaspoon almond extract
2   tablespoons almond butter
4   cups sliced strawberries, halved raspberries, blackberries,
       grapes, mandarin orange segments, or other fruit of
       your choice
    Fresh mint sprigs

In a large saucepan, whisk together soy milk, maple syrup, agar, and salt. Bring gradually to a boil over medium heat. Reduce heat and simmer uncovered until agar dissolves, about 5 minutes. Whisk occasionally.

Turn off heat and whisk in vanilla and almond extract. Pour into large bowl and cover with wax paper or plastic wrap to prevent skin from forming on top. Refrigerate 1½ hours to set.

When firm, add almond butter and blend until smooth. In six wine goblets, press sliced fruit against side of glass. Fill center with layers of almond cream and fruit.

Refrigerate until serving. Garnish with mint sprigs.

Yield: 6 servings

✖ FRESH PEACH COMPOTE
WITH ALMOND-ORANGE SYRUP

- ¼ teaspoon almond extract
- ½ cup orange juice
- ½ cup brown rice syrup or sorghum syrup
- Zest of 1 orange
- Zest of ¼ lemon
- A few grains of sea salt
- 2 pounds peaches (6 cups), peeled, halved, and cut into ½-inch slices, then in half crosswise
- ¼ cup sliced almonds, toasted and chopped
- Fresh mint sprigs

In a large bowl, whisk together all ingredients except peaches, almonds, and mint to make a syrup. Add peaches.

Serve immediately or (better still) allow compote to marinate. Serve fruit topped with syrup. Garnish with almonds and mint.

Note: A great deal of liquid comes out of the peaches as they marinate; this adds to the richness and volume of the compote. Stir occasionally as peaches are marinating for best results.

Yield: 6 servings

✄ STRAWBERRY SORBET

4   cups strawberries
½   cup maple syrup
1   tablespoon fresh lemon juice
½   cup soy milk
     Dash nutmeg

Put all ingredients in blender. Puree until smooth. Pour mixture into a freezer-proof container. Cover and freeze until sorbet is set (about 8½ hours).

Remove sorbet from the refrigerator and thaw for approximately 15 minutes. Break sorbet into 2-inch chunks with fork and puree again until smooth.

Return to container and freeze until mixture sets to desired texture (about 4 hours).

Yield: 4 to 6 servings

Skin Basics

~⌒

MOST OF US FORGET HOW SENSITIVE OUR SKIN IS TO TOUCH. INSTEAD, we believe that a few macho swipes with a towel or a slap of astringent lotion is enough to enrich our skin. Not so!

There is a reason why we are naturally drawn to cuddle and stroke babies. Their intellectual and social development actually requires a nurturing touch to grow healthy and to bond with others. Noted psychiatrist Karen Horney performed the landmark research on this issue several decades ago, and it still stands today. But the need for nurturing touch doesn't stop in infancy or even childhood. It is as important for adults as it is for the newborn.

To bring the nurturing, health-giving touch back into our adult lives, this chapter will show you how to massage your skin to encourage health and cellular repair. What's more, by lovingly applying creams and lotions, you will help your skin's acid mantle do the regenerative job nature intended.

By establishing a ritual of nurturing skin care, we develop an instant intimacy with—and responsibility for—our own anatomy. Doing so also allows us to start thanking our skin (and, indirectly, our entire body) for the good work it is doing. I promise you that, with regular care, your skin will glow and become as soft as a baby's bottom.

SKIN BASICS

Before proceeding with specific therapies and regimens, it is important to understand what the skin is and how it works. First, you should know that the skin is not only the "cover" that we present to the outside world, but, in an anatomical sense, the skin is our largest eliminatory and receptor organ and thus serves definite physiological purposes as well.

What exactly is the skin? It is a snug-fitting, protective barrier, composed of overlapping cells that shield our inner organs from unnecessary, possibly harmful contact with the outside world. At the same time, our skin selectively allows certain approved substances to enter our bodies through the pores and lets them into the inner workings of our cells. Without the skin's protective membrane, our inner cells would be at the absolute mercy of the elements—including fluctuations in temperature and all manner of diseases—while our vital fluids would be in a constant state of leakage and flux.

The skin is also our most vital organ of elimination. It continuously releases toxins produced by the inner cells, as well as water, through the pores. These pores serve as virtual doorways that open and close as required by internal processes. Among the toxins we release through the pores are uric acid, carbon dioxide, perspiration, dead bacteria, and invading live bacteria that cause illnesses. Interestingly, we also release what we eat through our pores, especially when we eat hot spices and herbs or drink liquor.

What neither the skin nor our bodies would ever want to release through the pores or membranes in large amounts is blood and lymph. Because doing so would constitute a life-threatening situation, the body constantly guards against this occurrence. When leakage does occur, by way of accident or intention (as in a surgical cut), an instant, intricate clotting mechanism is put into place.

KEEPING THE SKIN'S
ACID MANTLE HEALTHY

If you were to look the skin through a microscope, you might think you were viewing the craters of the moon—complete with living organisms! These actually are bacteria, viruses, worms, and/or parasites that claim squatting rights on our bodies.

Most of these organisms are harmless, but some are toxic; it is the skin's job to ensure that they are never allowed to enter the body. One of the mechanisms that the skin employs against inadvertent invasion is the secretion and maintenance of an acidic cover, called the acid mantle. This mantle is decidedly unfriendly toward unwelcome squatters and unhealthy outside chemicals and pollutants, and it also helps maintain the closed tone of the pores.

Obviously, it is extremely important to keep your skin's acid mantle in proper working order. You can do this by:

- lubricating your skin frequently with a friendly, nourishing moisturizer (see page 103)
- drinking enough plain (not carbonated) water every day
- adding approximately 2 tablespoons of uncooked, unrefined vegetable oil to your daily diet
- getting moderate amounts of daily outdoor exercise
- eating a healthy, balanced diet
- ensuring good bowel health

HOW ESSENTIAL OILS
HELP BEAUTIFY THE SKIN

The regular use of essential oils—in either creams, lotions, or blends—is the most natural and effective way you can keep your skin looking its best. In fact, using the essential oil blend that is best for your skin type can not only lubricate your skin but actually maintain its balance. Better news still is that essential oils can actually help repair the acid mantle.

In chapter 7, I provide a full range of treatments for specific skin woes that call upon essential oils to work the wonders for which they have been long known. How do we know our skin mantle balance is off-kilter? We get tip-offs in the form of excessive dryness or oiliness; scaly patches; and ulcers, dermatitis, psoriasis, and other skin ailments. All are messages that the skin cells and flesh in those areas are being degraded.

Happily, with proper essential oil lubrication, even these extreme imbalances can be corrected. I'll present the full range of treatments in chapter 7; but for now, you should know that my favorite skin-balancing oils are carrot, lavender, bergamot, rose, neroli, and benzoin, all used in a safflower oil base. For skin diseases, I use three of these essential oils followed by an application of a light avocado milky lotion or cream, reinforced with essential oils.

THE LONG HISTORY
OF ESSENTIAL OIL USE

Civilizations from ancient times have long known of the beautifying effects of essential oils. Such ancient texts as the Bible and Egyptian and North African writings all presented recipes with essential oils and botanical extracts. Many ancient civilizations had a tradition of using oils blended with flowers, resins, or other scented materials that were indigenous to their regions. For example, in India, sandalwood oil is routinely used in skin care. The women in North and Northeast Africa used myrrh or frankincense to help protect their skin from the rigors of a dry, harsh climate, while their Polynesian cousins were using coconut oil infused with gardenia blossoms for their regime. Meanwhile, in Peru, balsam was used for a wide array of skin care and other needs.

In Europe, essential oils have never gone out of style, and even mass-distributed products have long included various essential oils in their lists of ingredients. Women outside North America grow up learning that beauty is achieved from within (what we eat) and without (how we take care of our skin).

Interestingly, women in far-flung parts of the globe all learned to use essential oils to beautify their skins, just as they recognized the medicinal properties of plants of their regions to help maintain good health.

WHY ESSENTIAL OILS ARE BETTER

What women have known for centuries is finally being recognized. Aromatherapists are demonstrating essential oils' many curative properties and preventive actions, as well as the efficacy of essential oils diluted in vegetable oils as a building block to skin care.

Most people are unaware that complex chemicals in essential oils house nutritional compounds along with medicinal ingredients. Essential oils contain such micronutrients as calcium, magnesium, thiamin, riboflavin, potassium, carotene, iron, and zinc. By applying aromatherapy oils to the skin, these ingredients are absorbed by a process called tyransdermal absorption.

There is absolutely no comparison between a complexion nourished with aromatherapy blends and one congested with the mass-produced commercial creams and lotions most modern city women use. I consider most store-bought potions the "fast foods" of cosmetics. These creams and lotions are made mainly with fossil fuel (petrochemicals) and animal by-products, such as lanolin. The problem with these cosmetics is that petrochemicals, which come from long-dead materials, have the sluggish vibration that attracts dirt and clogs the pores. Petrochemicals, in their various adapted forms—mineral oil, baby oil, petroleum jelly, fragrances, alcohol, preservatives, etc.—are responsible for the vast majority of skin allergies today.

Animal by-products have different problems. Chief among these are spoilage, hence the need for preservatives (more petrochemicals!). Lanolin, the most commonly used by-product, is made by sheep to protect them from the weather. Lanolin, a fatty residue, coats the skin of the sheep, trapping heat and repelling water and cold. It was not meant to be absorbed into the body—either ours or the sheep's—but, rather, to be an effective insulation and barrier. Thus, while lanolin may have a place for women or men who work outdoors, it is not something most of us should be using every day, if at all.

Our skin is a clever protector all on its own. It prevents dirt and harmful invaders like bacteria from entering the body through its pores. In its healthy state, the skin is sealed fast against lipids, such as vegetable oils, animal fats, and petroleum oils. Only when the skin is wet and the pores are slightly dilated for respiration will the skin inadvertently allow dirt-bearing lipids through its pores. When this happens, it is as a result of the dilated pores closing back around the oil molecules lying on the wet skin.

Just imagine—this is the main selling point of products like baby oil and Vaseline as moisturizers! Corporate marketers try to convince us that we should use these products on our bodies after showering because our wet skin might be persuaded to absorb some of these lipids. The skin, in its infinite natural wisdom, would never allow baby oil into the body because of its potential ability to carry harmful bacteria inside after the skin has dried.

Essential oil blends, on the other hand, are recognized by the skin as the healthy, clean, life-affirming aids that they are. Proof positive: We don't have to fool the skin by applying essential oils only when the skin is wet. Our skin's pores open up willingly when essential oils knock on the door. This is so because not only are the essential oil molecules extremely tiny and vibrant, but they also have the intensely high vibration of *amplified* life—which is closely akin to the highest vibration of all, the spiritual vibration.

This intense power of essential oils is passed on to the vegetable oil matrix of aromatherapy blends. Essential oils actually change the molecular structure of the vegetable oils into which they are blended to make the resulting compound more acceptable to the skin.

CHAPTER 7

ESSENTIAL BEAUTY ROUTINES

~⁀

NOW FOR THE ESSENTIAL BEAUTY ROUTINES THAT WILL HAVE YOU looking and feeling better than you ever dreamed—regardless of your age, skin type, and the present condition of your skin. In fact, if your skin is not quite as beautiful as it should be, you will notice the dramatic results in your complexion all the faster.

The first thing we should realize is that unlike many other animals, human beings don't have fur or other protective body covering. It is for this reason that we have had to find coverings for our own skin, from the animal hides of Stone Age days to the Spandex fashions of our own time. With good reason: Our skin is among the most delicate and thin of all mammals.

However, despite its vulnerability to the environment, our skin is remarkably resilient. It is amazingly efficient as a protective cover for our inner organs, its primary function. Still, our skin does need consistent help from us to do its work properly. It cannot function optimally without proper nutrition *inside* and *outside*.

The simple act of drinking six to eight glasses of water a day, as previously mentioned, goes a great distance toward helping our skin create and maintain its acid mantle covering from the inside. That, plus a balanced diet, is more than half the battle won. We can also treat our skin from the outside, as this chapter will detail. Using the right moisturizers on the skin's surface helps the skin to maintain and nourish the acid mantle from the outside. This, then, is a two-tiered program whose beautiful results are very much more than the sum of their parts.

WHAT'S THE SCOOP ON THE SUN?

Just as North Americans have been taught to demonize much of the food we eat, so too are we being taught to hate the sun. The potential for skin damage is a real concern, of course, but it's not the sun's fault. Because the industrial age has succeeded in destroying a good portion of the protective etheric skin of the Earth—also known as the ozone layer—our scientists have blamed the sun itself, the very body that gives us life. The real problem is unhealthy living and a disrespect for the Earth. We have shot off more harmful chemicals into the air in the last century than had been done in hundreds of thousands of years prior to the Industrial Revolution. Then, we try to blame the sun—how dare it be so hot! If we keep using petrochemicals and eating salt- and chemical-laden fast food, we will all become hotter still, because these items, by their very nature, combine to give us a suffocating, overheated feeling. Moreover, the more we manufacture and use synthetic materials, the greater the hole in the ozone, and the hotter the sun will get.

Rather than demonize it, why not start celebrating the sun? It supplies us with hard-to-get vitamin D when we soak in its rays, along with that incomparable feeling of upliftment, serenity, and joy. It is hard to imagine real health and beauty without a few minutes in the natural sunshine, along with copious amounts of fresh air. Just remember to limit your exposure (even with the natural sunscreen effects of the essential oils); during the day's warmest hours, admire the sun from afar—in the shade.

What About Sunscreens?

Ten years ago, nobody talked about sunscreen in moisturizers. Today, it's the big buzzword; no product is worth its weight unless it contains sunscreen in addition to all its other miracle ingredients.

I would never suggest that you give up the sunscreen that you are most comfortable with, especially if it contains mainly healthy, skin-friendly botanical ingredients. That said, I would strongly suggest that you add essential oils to your present protective regimen. The essential oils I present in my skin care regimens contain natural sunscreen properties that help protect against sun damage and, in some cases, can even help repair the skin.

There's another big plus to using essential oils. Because they help clean up the air, the more we use them, the more we will be helping the environment around us to stay healthy and fresh. This happens because the molecules in essential oils actually destroy pollution and other toxins as they evaporate up and out into the air.

There are some commonsense pointers we should all follow when going out in the sun. These include:

- avoiding the sun during the hottest part of the day for extended periods, if at all possible
- wearing sun protectors (hats, glasses, visors) when out in the sun
- using essential oils to lubricate and balance the skin and to help protect against skin damage

OTHER SKIN ADVICE

Apart from how we relate to the sun, if I had to give just one other piece of advice, it would be this: Never—and I mean never—wear your makeup to bed. And I mean all makeup—foundation, powder (especially tinted powder), mascara, blush, and anything else. Most traumatizing to the skin is foundation, because it blocks the pores and keeps dirt virtually trapped on the skin. So, at a time when your pores should be open and respirating properly on clean skin, you instead have a suffocating cover that is preventing the release and removal of toxins. Moreover, foundation prohibits the generation of healthy new cells and actually promotes the inadvertent overstimulation of the oil-producing sebaceous glands in the dermis that lies below the outer skin.

When I was younger, more foolish, and more fearlessly pursuing beauty at all costs, I would make the common mistake of applying foundation and powder to my oily/combination skin. In so doing, I was trying (futilely!) to replicate the smooth, matte look that was popular at the time. Of course, the more I applied foundation and powder, the more the natural shine on my face would appear, even after just a couple of hours. I even tried applying cold packs to my finished makeup—and while the immediate response was gratifying, the long-term results were much less so.

Although my complexion was always basically attractive, I had the slight problem that many black- and brown-skinned women have—a darker blotchiness around the chin and cheeks, which were habitually drier than the skin on my forehead and nose. By trying to even out the various brown tones, I actually exacerbated the very condition I was trying to correct.

The good news was that when I started studying skin care and facial anatomy, I found that by giving myself regular facials with essential oils, I helped even out my skin tone naturally. Today, I only wear makeup when I appear on television, at the requirement of the show's producers. Even though I always make a point of asking for sensitive-skin, hypoallergenic, theatrical makeup, it can be agony after a couple of hours. With this war paint on, my eyes start to swell up, get red, and tear, and my skin breaks out in itchy blotches, especially in the cheeks and on the temples. How do people wear this stuff every day?

THE BENEFITS OF AROMATHERAPY FACIALS

I have given countless aromatherapy facials to virtually every skin type and on men and women of all ages. Even when skin was so discolored that it looked like calico or so sun-damaged that it was flushed and leathery, the typical, immediate, amazed response after an aromatherapy facial might be the following:

- Did you just get cosmetic surgery?
- Did you have your face planed?
- You look fabulous—are you in love?

If you take the time to develop a healthy regimen, people may soon start asking you these very questions. So let's jump right in with the basics.

THE BEST BEAUTY ROUTINE
FOR YOUR SKIN TYPE

Given the proliferation of products on the market, it is hardly surprising that even hyperintelligent women are at sea when it comes to selecting an ongoing beauty routine. I have one client, an MBA who runs a huge division of a multinational company, who recently implored, "Help me, Pat! I don't have a clue what to use on my face every day!"

Little wonder, with the seemingly endless array of commercial products available. Just one look at the advertising pages of major women's magazines is enough to make any woman dizzy. Yet all of us modern women are potential victims of advertising. The trick is to utter a resounding "no!" Just as you will now reject all the TV and print ads for fake food products, so, too, will you know not to be seduced by the creams and potions nineteen-year-old models try to get us to buy. Just banning these products from your bathroom shelf—and credit card bills—should do much to put a smile on your face. As Joni Mitchell sang, "Happiness is the best face-lift." Indeed!

Establishing a good skin care regimen can be easy, supplemented by just a little bit of common sense and action. Remember: Not only do we want our skin to look better, but by following the suggestions in this book, you will also help your skin to *be* better as it begins to function more efficiently in its dual role of protector and detox filter of the inner organs of your body.

Determining Your Skin Type

This is the $64 million question and the area in which many women go painfully, dreadfully wrong. In fact, I would estimate that a full half of my new clients are not only using damaging commercial products but have also had a poorly trained beauty "expert" behind the cosmetics counter at their local department store utterly and totally misdiagnose their skin type.

In botany, we consider the flower to be the face of the plant, with the plant presenting this face upward, glorifying the sun and flirting with the pollinator. Flowers definitely compete with each other to call their pollinators to themselves, and that is why we have such a dazzling variety of beautiful colors and scents.

In our human world, I like to think of our faces as the flowers we present to the sun and the outside world, offering up as many varieties of beauty and color as our botanical counterparts.

Now, with the perfect fusion of man and nature, we can use nature's bounty to enhance our own health and beauty.

Let's consider the various complexion types.

- fair, sensitive skin; often, with broken capillaries or "couperose" over the nose and/or cheeks; ruddy color, sometimes with acne rosacea
- fair, dry, thin skin; beautiful when younger, quickest to age
- mottled, discolored skin; oily, acne-prone, with open pores (usually associated with teenagers)
- mottled, discolored skin; mature type
- sensitive skin; olive and dark
- mature, with wrinkles and sagging jowls
- ashen black skin, easily scarred or discolored
- combination skin; any genetic type
- oily/normal combination skin type

The extensive range suggested above can be simplified into several main areas:

1. mature/wrinkled/dry
2. sensitive
3. sun damaged
4. oily/acne rosacea
5. dull, lifeless skin (including ashy black skin)

THE BEST ESSENTIAL OILS FOR YOUR SKIN TYPE

Essential oils blended in combinations for your skin type or special needs can become the best friend your complexion might ever need. Listed below are some suggestions for at-home care or salon use. Regular use of aromatherapy oils can help to ward off the aging process, balance oiliness or excessive dryness, even out skin tone and discolorations, and protect against the elements. In general, the sweet florals, combined with either citruses or woods, can have an extremely beautifying effect on the skin.

ACNE: Bay, lavender, lemongrass, jasmine, juniper, tangerine, ylang-ylang

DRY SKIN: Chamomile, geranium, neroli, orange, myrrh, rose, sandalwood

COUPEROSE: Chamomile, carrot, geranium, sandalwood

SENSITIVE SKIN: Chamomile, lavender, neroli, patchouli, rosewood

MUSCLE TONE: Cypress, jasmine, frankincense, lemon, sandalwood

HAIR CONDITIONING: Bay, bergamot, chamomile, geranium, rosemary, sage, thyme

FROWN LINES: Carrot, frankincense, myrrh, neroli, sandalwood

EYE CARE: Lavender water, chamomile water, rose water; Oils: Chamomile, carrot, lavender, rosemary (to reduce bags)

SUN-DAMAGED, LEATHERY, OR MATURE SKIN: Bergamot, carrot, cedarwood, frankincense, lavender, myrrh, neroli, patchouli, rosewood, sandalwood

DÉCOLLETAGE: Orange, myrrh, rose, pettigrain, pine, tangerine, ylang-ylang

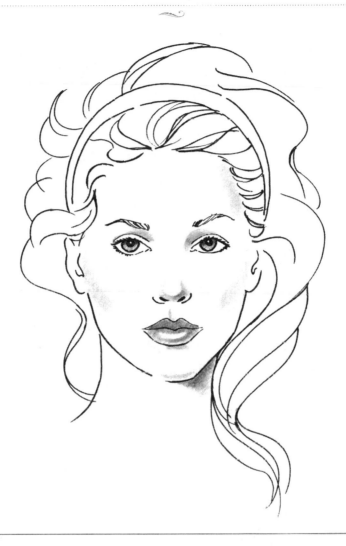

For best facial care, prevention is the key. Start using natural, synthetic-free, plant-extract products, lotions, and masks, along with aromatherapy combination oils based on your skin type, seasons, emotions, or other needs. Exfoliation is a must for all skin types to ensure proper turnover of healthy young cells. This should be followed up by toning and nourishing. Even skins that have lost elasticity and are dehydrated can become radiantly improved in a very short time.

Most adults have combination-type complexions, whether it is normal/dry, or oily T-zone (forehead, nose, chin), or dry/sensitive. However, to simplify matters, choose which of the five categories on page 97 most closely describes your skin.

Quite frankly, so-called normal skin, the coveted, even-textured, creamy, smooth, poreless look that many of us crave, is almost a myth among adult women (or men). It is actually found almost exclusively on babies and small children! Our mission, in seeking skin health and beauty, is to bring every skin type as close to "normal" as possible, given your age and genetic and complexion type.

DAILY BEAUTY ESSENTIALS

There are three easy-to-remember steps to good skin care and health:

1. cleanse
2. tone
3. moisturize

Cleansing

Although some complexion types respond well to a good soap-and-water wash every day, most of us—especially women over the age of twenty-five—do not. So we may have to use creams or lotions to cleanse, followed by a clean water rinse afterward.

Most commercial facial cleansers should be avoided, especially if they contain mineral oil as their primary ingredient. Mineral oil, as stated earlier, is a petrochemical that suffocates the skin as it leaches through the pores.

In fact, cleansing your facial skin is not as important as you might think, unless you routinely use skin-clogging foundation and makeup. (Does that make me sound like some kind of a revolutionary—or worse yet, a heretic?) The reason is this: Toning, which is essential for everyone, is actually more important. The exception is if you have oily skin, which I discuss in the section starting on page 112.

If you feel compelled to wash your face in the morning (but please, never twice a day!), buy your cleanser not in the drugstore or at a fancy department store counter but in a reputable health food store or through aromatherapy suppliers, like those in the Resource Guide at the end of this book. Look for products whose main ingredient is a plant or vegetable oil or water.

To use these cleansers, apply the product to a moist cotton pad (warm water is best). Apply to the skin. Rinse first with warm water, which rids the skin of oil, then pat with cool water and tone immediately thereafter.

Toning

In my opinion, toning is the most important of the three steps. Sadly, in this country, it is the one most often skipped. We tone when we apply a liquid, slightly acidic fluid, such as witch hazel, to our skin. *Never* use alcohol as a toner—even if you have oily skin; over the long term, harsh alcohols destroy the skin.

Toning your face every day with a good floral water or floral vinegar quickly removes the cleansing residue from your skin, removing impurities that cleansing has left behind. Even more important, a good toner will restore the skin's acid mantle, a requisite to good looks and health.

How to use a toner is also a matter of some concern. I have seen many women who literally douse a cotton ball with toner and leave their faces sopping wet! This is bad enough when one uses the right kind of toner, but when a woman uses the superdrying alcohol-based products that are commercially available, the results can be devastating to the skin. In this case, it's much better not to tone at all. The correct way to use a toner follows:

1. Dampen a cotton pad with cool water.
2. Squeeze excess water out of the pad.
3. Put just a few drops of toner on the pad.
4. Wipe the face with it in circles.
5. Tone your face both morning and night, before moisturizing.

Moisturizing

Absolutely mandatory! The trick, of course, is to find the right moisturizer for your skin type and complexion needs. This is where the personalization of the essential oils becomes de rigueur.

The toner and moisturizer that are best for your skin type are listed in the categories that follow.

MATURE/WRINKLED SKIN

Many years ago, a woman came to me for aromatherapy advice. She was obviously older, a feisty, slender person in good health and with good eating habits. I put her biological age at about seventy and marveled at the stamina that she obviously enjoyed. We worked out a simple skin-care regimen that she was to start right away. She had thin, extremely wrinkled, and sun-damaged mature skin. The skin around her neck was sagging and soft. This woman was obviously a combination of types.

I made her a myrrh oil compound (see page 106) and advised her to use it twice a day. I also recommended that she have a monthly facial. Although she only allowed herself three facials a year, she was quite faithful in her use of the myrrh oil. After about a year, I saw her again, and her skin was much improved. Thirteen years later, I had the opportunity to examine her again. To my astonishment, I realized that she was not seventy when we first met

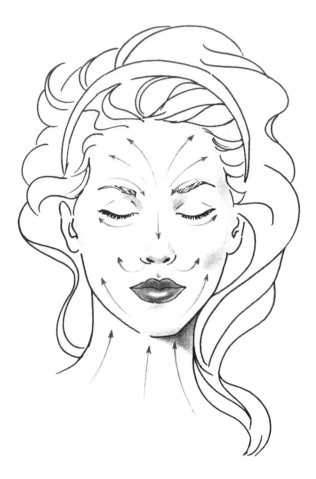

🐚 FACIAL MASSAGE

Step 1 Pour ½ capful of aromatherapy oil into your palm; apply all over your face and neck and begin your massage.

1. Starting at chin, stroke upward and outward, following direction of arrows.

2. Circle around eyes with middle finger.

3. Stroke forehead upward and outward to lift and help eliminate fine lines. Repeat this sequence at least three more times.

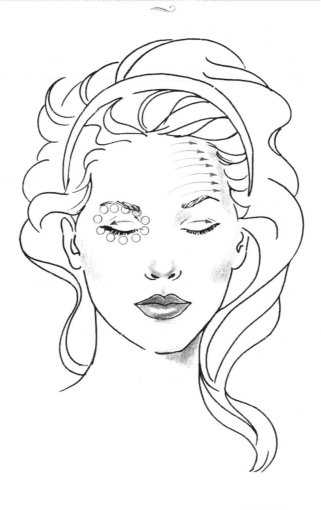

Step 2 After initial massage (see Step 1), apply pressure point strokes.

1. With thumbs, apply firm pressure, holding for a couple seconds on the eye socket bone, following circles around the eye. Do not apply these pressure strokes on the thin, loose skin of the eyelids. Apply pressure only on eyebrows and on bone below lower lids.

2. Lightly stroke eyelids with cream or oil.

because she told me that this was her age now. You do the math: This means that she was only in her fifties when we first met! Her wrinkled skin added almost twenty years to her appearance.

This is a truly dramatic example of how essential oils can rejuvenate even mature damaged skin to an amazing degree. This seventy-year-old client's skin is now smooth and barely wrinkled—even around the neck—with a youthful glow emanating from below the surface of the skin.

Toner

Rose water or neroli water are the best toners for mature or wrinkled skin. They are available at health food stores (or check the Resource Guide in the back of this book).

Moisturizer

MYRRH OIL COMPOUND

    40 drops myrrh oil
    40 drops ylang-ylang oil
    10 drops neroli oil
    10 drops cypress oil
    20 drops sweet orange oil
     1 ounce safflower or grapeseed oil

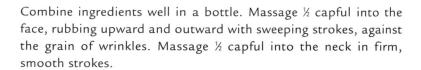

Combine ingredients well in a bottle. Massage ½ capful into the face, rubbing upward and outward with sweeping strokes, against the grain of wrinkles. Massage ½ capful into the neck in firm, smooth strokes.

Nightly, smooth in your favorite all-natural botanical cream (from any good health food or aromatherapy store) over the oil.

Mask

SUPERFIRMING MASK

¼   cup plain yogurt

2   teaspoons brewer's yeast or Missing Link powder

1   drop geranium oil

½   teaspoon fruit vinegar

1   drop rose oil

1   tablespoon wheat germ oil

Combine all ingredients in a small bowl. Spread thickly over face and neck. Leave on for 20 minutes. While you are doing the mask, cover your eyes with cotton pads soaked in diluted rose water. Before removing the mask, spritz face with rose water. After 2 minutes, rinse off well and tone with rose water. Use this toning mask once a month.

SENSITIVE SKIN

Those of you with sensitive skin already know that your skin type requires special attention. In my experience, an aromatherapy-based skin-care regimen is especially helpful for this kind of skin, because it is the type most easily damaged by harsh commercial products.

Toner

Lavender water or neroli water are the best toners for sensitive skin. Use twice daily.

Moisturizer

CHAMOMILE MOISTURIZING OIL

30 drops blue chamomile oil
10 drops lavender oil
10 drops rosewood oil
10 drops patchouli oil
 5 drops bergamot oil
 1 ounce avocado oil

Combine all ingredients in a bottle. Shake well to blend. Massage a small amount into face and neck, using upward and outward strokes on the face, and downward and outward circles and strokes for the neck.

Nighttime Moisturizer

Buy an aloe gel puree that is more liquid than viscous at a health food store. Add 1 teaspoon lavender water to 2 ounces of this gel mixture for a wonderful nighttime moisturizer for even the most sensitive skins. Nightly, pat this mixture over the skin.

Mask

BEAUTIFYING BOTANICAL MASK

½   cup pureed cucumbers
1   teaspoon dried milk powder
1   drop lavender oil
½   teaspoon rose hip–seed oil

Mix all ingredients into a thick paste in a wooden bowl. Apply thickly to the face and neck. Leave on for 15 minutes. Rinse off and tone with lavender water. Apply moisturizing oil or gel.

Use this mask once a month to improve the look of sensitive skin.

SUN-DAMAGED SKIN

Whenever I look at cowboys on film (having grown up in Jamaica, I have a soft spot for old American Westerns!), I am appalled by the sun damage I see. The cowboy's skin is so weathered and leathery.

As much as I respect and honor the sun, I see almost daily how much damage can be wreaked on unprotected or dry skin. The skin literally turns to leather on some people. So, if any cowboys (or girls) are reading this book, you may want to try the regimen I have created especially for you.

"Cowboy skin" typically is dehydrated, flaky, taut, and deeply lined around the eyes and mouth. It is also mottled in appearance, with discolored patches all around.

Toner

Rose water or fruit vinegar (see Resource Guide) are the best toners for sun-damaged skin.

Moisturizer

✍ CARROT OIL COMPOUND

30 drops carrot seed oil
20 drops rose oil
20 drops bergamot oil
30 drops frankincense oil
20 drops lavender oil
2 teaspoons evening primrose oil
1 tablespoon jojoba oil
2 ounces grapeseed oil

Mix all ingredients well in a bottle. Massage into face and neck using sweeping, circular movements. Do this twice a day.

Mask

PAPAYA MASK

¼ cup papaya puree (available at health food stores)
2 tablespoons heavy cream
½ teaspoon arrowroot powder
2 drops chamomile oil

Mix all ingredients in a small bowl until smooth. Apply thickly to face and neck. Leave on for 20 minutes. Rinse off and tone with lavender water.

Use this mask twice monthly to help reverse the effects of skin damage.

Extra tip for sun-damaged skin: If you use lavender water or diluted fruit vinegar to cleanse your face (instead of a vegetable or plant oil–based product, as for other skin types), you will help to restore the acid mantle to your skin. This is especially important for sun-damaged skin.

Tip for anyone out in the sun: To quickly cool off when outdoors, just spritz your skin and head with lavender water. This is a great skin preserver whether you work outdoors, are sunbathing, or just happen to be taking an extended stroll in the heat.

OILY/ACNE-PRONE SKIN

Oily/acne-prone skin tends to be young, while acne rosacea skin (which follows) tends to occur on more mature skins. Both are what I would call a "hot" condition. By this, I mean that the skin tends to be hot to begin with, then heats up even more with certain physical or chemical stresses. These can be climatic or the result of using chemically imbalanced skin-care products and cosmetics. Those outbreaks can happen all year round and tend to be exacerbated during the summer, since the skin becomes more oily when the weather is humid and hot.

There is a silver lining to this cloud, however, and a very nice one at that! The good news about oily skin is that it remains young looking throughout a woman's life. On the other hand, the bad news is that the clogging of the sebum cells leads to acne, open pores, and breakouts, which are not so lovely.

Most women with oily skin types tend to use too many drying products. As explained earlier, this leads to even more surface oil and blockages. This is the skin type that reaps the most rewards from conscientious washing and water-based cleansing.

Cleansing and Toning

If you have oily skin, you should disregard the general cleansing procedure I outlined earlier. Instead:

1. Wash your face with olive oil soap twice daily.
2. Tone with lavender water or neroli water at least three times a day, especially during the summer months.
3. Use a balancing light cream every morning. (In hot weather, essential oils in vegetable oils heat up the skin too much, which is why I am recommending a light cream instead.)

Moisturizing

✍ BALANCING LIGHT CREAM

2 ounces vegetable oil cream (available in health food stores or see the Resource Guide in the back of the book)
1 teaspoon lavender water
1 teaspoon cornstarch or arrowroot powder
5 drops ylang-ylang oil
5 drops bay oil
5 drops lavender oil

Combine all ingredients in a bowl. Blend until smooth and creamy. Keep refrigerated in a plastic jar.

Apply twice daily by lightly stroking over face and neck.

Mask

✏ BALANCING MASK

- 2 tablespoons honey
- 1 ounce ground adzuki beans or powdered oatmeal
- 1 teaspoon lemon juice
- ½ egg white

Combine all ingredients in a small bowl until a paste forms. Apply over clean skin and let set for 30 minutes. Rinse well with warm water, using washcloth if necessary. Afterward, tone with lavender water.

Use this balancing mask once a week.

Exfoliant

This is the only skin type for which I recommend a specific exfoliant. It is extremely important that oily-skinned women exfoliate to remove the top cells of their skin. Other skin types can benefit from exfoliation as well. For the simplest at-home exfoliation, simply rub a washcloth, dampened with the toner for your specific skin type, in small, circular movements all over your face.

OILY SKIN EXFOLIANT

2   teaspoons granulated sugar
1   tablespoon olive oil
2   drops lemon oil

Mix in a small bowl just before using. The sugar grains should not be liquid.

Apply to skin in circular movements all over face and neck. Rinse off with warm water and remove oil with lavender toner on cotton pads.

Special tip for oily/acne rosacea skin: Use only cornstarch or arrowroot as a face powder. Never use a liquid, tinted foundation. Instead, use a water-based, clear foundation when necessary.

ACNE ROSACEA-PRONE SKIN

Like oily skin, those with rosacea have skin that tends to heat up quickly.

Toner

Use lavender water as a toner at least twice a day.

Moisturizer

✐ CHAMOMILE LEMON LAVENDER CREAM

2   ounces vegetable oil cream
10   drops blue chamomile oil
5   drops lemon oil
5   drops lavender oil
1   teaspoon arrowroot powder

Combine all ingredients in a bowl until smooth. Lightly massage small amounts into face and neck.

Soak a washcloth in cold water with ice cubes added; wring out. Gently pat over face and neck. Blot dry and pat with a tissue.

Mask

✐ HONEY GEL MASK

1   cup aloe gel or seaweed gel (from health food store)
1   tablespoon honey
1   tablespoon lavender water
1   tablespoon papaya puree (from health food store)

Combine all ingredients in a bowl and apply thickly to face and neck, refrigerating the leftover paste in a plastic container. Leave on for 20 minutes. Rinse off. Tone with lavender water.

DULL, LIFELESS, OR ASHY BLACK SKIN

Black skin looks ashy when it is overly dehydrated and/or lacking in oxygen. Two of the greatest culprits are harsh astringents and heavy foundation or powder. All skin needs to breathe as a prerequisite to proper regeneration. Most important, stop using harsh cleansers and astringents immediately!

In addition, it is important to watch your diet carefully. Make sure you are not overloading on fried foods and simple carbohydrates. The healthy diet regimens we described earlier, plus extra water (at least six to eight glasses a day is best) are important steps in taking care of your skin and your health.

One of my assistants came to me years ago because of problems with her skin. She had been misdiagnosed by top salons as having thick, oily skin when, in fact, she had thin, dehydrated, and (as is often the case with black skin) very sensitive skin. Alas, her face looked like a lifeless mask.

I recommended a cleansing and rejuvenating facial. Even with just one treatment, her beautiful clear skin began to emerge. After a few sessions more, she looked like a new woman. With the regular use of essential oils (and the treatments listed below), her skin glows like an orchid!

Cleanser

Cleanse your skin with a light cleansing lotion such as Aubrey Organics (available at health food stores and at some pharmacies). Be sure to cleanse morning and night.

Toner

Tone your skin twice daily with rose water.

Moisturizer

GRAPEFRUIT OIL PLUS

    10   drops rose oil
    10   drops carrot seed oil
    20   drops grapefruit oil
    10   drops benzoin oil
    ½   ounce rose hip–seed oil
    ½   ounce rice bran oil
    ½   ounce avocado oil

Combine all ingredients in a bottle and blend well. Massage in firm upward and outward strokes on face; use downward and outward strokes on the neck, for 5 minutes each.

Blot skin with clean, white tissue.

Exfoliant

Exfoliation is extremely important for ashy black skin. This is because by constantly removing the dull, lifeless surface skin cells, the newly forming cells in the dermis are supplied with the stimulation and oxygen that they need.

PAPAYA MUSH EXFOLIATOR

½   cup papaya puree (available in health food stores)
1   tablespoon Missing Link powder or brewer's yeast
1   drop lemon oil

Combine all ingredients in a small bowl until a paste is formed. Spread thickly over face and neck; leave on for 30 minutes. Rinse well, first with a dampened face cloth, then with plain water. Tone with rose water. Use this treatment once a week.

CHAPTER 8

OTHER RECIPES FOR BEAUTY

THE EYES

 BRIGHT EYES NATURAL LID DEPUFFER

Those models who use Preparation H under their eyes after a night of hard partying would do much better to use this organically based preparation that I have personally used for years.

    5   drops chamomile essential oil
    5   drops lavender essential oil
    3   drops carrot essential oil
    2   tablespoons safflower oil

Mix all ingredients in a small bottle. To make puffy eyes disappear, dot around eye area sparingly at bedtime. If used regularly, this delightful blend will help to relieve dark circles and puffiness.

HAND AND FOOT CARE

Unless we get frequent manicures and pedicures, most of us just don't pamper our hands and feet enough. When we don't properly care for our feet, the result is dry, cracked skin with calluses, corns, and thickened ridges. On uncared-for hands, the skin becomes dry, thinner, and mottled or discolored.

This is not a natural part of aging; rather, it is the direct result of not caring for your extremities, specifically, not adequately moisturizing the hands and feet.

Let me give you an example. Many years ago, I did volunteer work at a senior citizen center in New York City. Everyone looked pretty much as you would expect, except Mrs. Smith. A woman of about eighty years old, she was definitely the glamour girl of the bunch! She had the most beautiful skin and always turned up with her short hair nicely but simply styled, with flattering makeup in place. However, the truly amazing thing about her was her hands. Mrs. Smith had alabaster skin, smooth and satiny, with no discernible age spots of any kind. It turned out that she had been a hand model when she was young and had learned to take care of her hands and skin as a matter of daily routine. When the other residents wanted cookies or sweets for their prizes (contests were de rigueur), Mrs. Smith only wanted the moisturizers, rose petal soaps, or floral waters I'd brought as her bounty. Smart lady—and a very pretty one, too!

SIMPLE HAND/FOOT OIL

20 drops carrot seed oil
10 drops lemon oil
10 drops rose oil
10 drops myrrh oil
½ ounce camellia or grapeseed oil

Combine all ingredients in a ½-ounce bottle and mix well. Massage 1 capful of resulting blend into hands and feet every day.

Alternatively, buy a vegetable oil botanical cream from the health food store. Blend 2 capfuls of the above essential oil mixture into 2 ounces cream, and massage into hands and feet regularly.

NAIL FUNGUS

Twenty years ago, when I first began my work, I didn't know *anyone* with nail fungus. But now, it seems to have reached nearly epidemic proportions. Possible culprits include unhealthy eating habits, improper hygiene, chemical poisoning, synthetic fibers, and acid mantle imbalance. I suspect there are many contributors to the proliferation of nail fungus, but I do know that using essential oils—especially lemon, pine, thyme, clove, geranium, and tea tree—along with a detoxifying diet can help to quickly remedy this problem.

To apply essential oils to the fungus, use only undiluted essential oils, applied with a Q-tip or eyedropper directly onto the affected nail(s). Put the oil under the nail, over it, and on the cuticle area as well. I suggest alternating pure lemon oil and pure tea tree oil.

In addition, massage a combination of aromatherapy blends into your hands and feet every day. This supplies proper nutrition to the cells and helps restore a balanced acid mantle to the area.

At least three times a week, soak the infected area in a hand and/or foot bath of warm water, as follows:

ANTIFUNGAL HAND AND FOOT BATH

```
 5  drops lemon oil
10  drops clove oil
 5  drops geranium oil
```

To a warm-to-hot hand or foot bath, add the above ingredients and stir to mix. Enjoy the fragrant scents as the oils' healing properties attack the fungus on your nails. Keep the fungal area immersed for about 15 minutes, 3 times a week.

CELLULITE

Cellulite appears as bumpy, puffy, soft, dimpled masses underneath the surface of the skin. On women, it most commonly shows up on the thighs, stomach, buttocks, and upper arms.

The most common causes of cellulite are:

- toxic debris trapped in the tissue spaces
- poor eating habits
- malnutrition
- excess consumption of salt and sugar
- lack of proper exercise
- sluggish digestion
- poor circulation, especially lymphatic circulation
- hormone imbalances
- repeated use of antibiotics and other drugs
- overexposure to insecticides

How to Get Rid of Cellulite

Exercise

A disciplined exercise program is the first step to take. This should include lots of stretches, particularly yoga and ballet-type stretches, which are actually more effective (contrary to popular opinion) than heavy weights or aerobic activity.

Nutrition

Healthy eating habits, like the ones outlined earlier in this book, can also help reduce cellulite. A diet rich in vegetables and other whole foods will help release toxins and improve all the operating systems of the body. Conversely, processed foods laced with preservatives and chemicals will have the opposite effect.

Essential Oils for Massage

Massage and spa treatments are also very effective, but only if they are followed consistently. The use of essential oils as part of these routines make these treatments even more efficacious, with even more dramatic results.

I suggest the following essential oils for massage therapy:

- cypress
- fennel
- juniper
- lemon
- lime
- grapefruit
- patchouli
- rosemary
- sassafras
- sage

In cellulite treatments, we aim to drain the lymphatic system and stimulate the circulation of blood throughout the body. During massage of the leg, it is very important to rub the thigh in upward, circular, kneading movements toward the groin area and lymph nodes. When massaging the arms, raise the upper arms above the head and massage downward, toward the armpit and lymph nodes in that area.

Massage each area with your aromatherapy blend for approximately 5 minutes. Do this every day, and you will begin to notice a firming and smoothing of the tissue. Massage each area briskly.

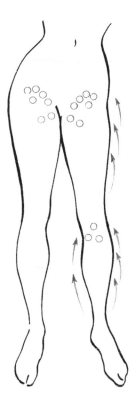

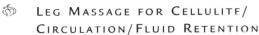

LEG MASSAGE FOR CELLULITE/ CIRCULATION/FLUID RETENTION

1. Pour 1 capful aromatherapy blend into palms.

2. Stroke the legs in upward movements, beginning at ankles and working toward knees.

3. Apply slightly deeper pressure on calf muscle, ending inside knee (where the lymph nodes are located).

4. Apply deep strokes from knee up to thighs toward groin area and lymph nodes.

5. Make strokes deeper and faster all over thighs, up to lymph nodes again.

6. Repeat sequence 4 times.

🍃 CELLULITE ESSENTIAL OIL TREATMENT

30 drops lemon essential oil
20 drops grapefruit essential oil
20 drops juniper essential oil
20 drops patchouli essential oil
10 drops clary sage essential oil
    Grapeseed oil

Pour essential oils into a 1-ounce bottle. Add enough grapeseed oil to fill the bottle. Blend well.

Use this blend every day as a massage oil on affected areas, massaging well for about 5 minutes on each area.

CIRCULATION PROBLEMS

Puffy Ankles/Fluid Retention

Sometimes we retain excess fluid in certain body parts. This can be the result of many factors or conditions, including:

- overweight
- hormone fluctuation
- salty diet
- travel

Once again, essential oils can provide much relief. All essential oils are diuretics, some more than others. Given this property, they will speedily break up fluid blockages and direct their healing properties to circulation and elimination organs. The end result of this redirection is more frequent urination—and, in some cases, more perspiration as well. Thus, essential oils can help to keep fluid moving around in the body as it was always meant to do.

❦ SIMPLE FLUID RETENTION OIL

10 drops fennel essential oil
20 drops lime essential oil
10 drops geranium essential oil
    Safflower oil

Put all essential oils into a ½-ounce bottle. Add enough safflower oil to fill bottle and mix well.

For puffy ankles: Massage in circles around the ankles and feet and up the lower calf with fingertips for 5 minutes on each leg.

For puffy tummy: Rub tummy with the flat part of your hand in clockwise circles. Start with wide circles, pressing firmly; then narrow the circles down around the navel. Go back to wide circles around larger area and repeat sequence for about 5 minutes.

Some people experience gas and/or gurgling sounds when they give themselves this massage. Don't be alarmed; you are just getting things moving, and the puffiness will soon abate.

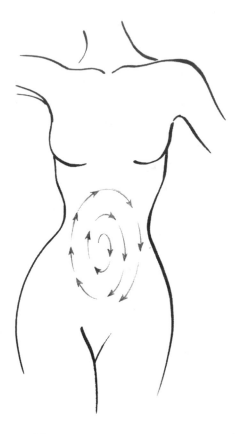

ABDOMINAL MASSAGE

Good for digestion, weight reduction, relaxation, and menstrual cramps.

1. Pour 1 capful of aromatherapy blend into palms and rub together.

2. Smooth oil over tummy for a couple minutes.

3. Starting near navel, work fingertips in small to larger circles, going from right side of tummy to left.

4. End strokes at base of lower left tummy.

Repeat sequence 3 times.

❧ ROSEMARY LEG REVITALIZER

For centuries, rosemary's rejuvenative powers have been celebrated. This oil works wonders on all manner of leg problems, from puffy ankles to cellulite to just plain tired legs. Many of my clients who work on their feet all day would not be without this revitalizing solution; it's also a must for tourists or anyone else who loves to walk, hike, or jog.

20   drops rosemary essential oil
10   drops cypress essential oil
10   drops geranium essential oil
15   drops fennel essential oil
½   ounce olive oil
½   ounce refined castor oil

Combine all ingredients in a glass bottle. (You can easily use a salad shaker with a snap-tight top.) Massage a small amount of oil into your feet and ankles, or over the entire leg if you suffer from cellulite. In this case, you should massage the oils over your legs in an upward, circular motion for 5 minutes. It feels even better if you can get a mate or friend to do it! Then relax with your feet and legs elevated for at least 10 minutes.

THE HAIR

How can essential oils help keep your hair healthy and beautiful? Let me count the ways! Some essential oils condition the hair, while others can eliminate dandruff, seborrhea, and/or dermatitis. Others will encourage hair growth (or regrowth, in the case of hair that has been lost due to chemotherapy or male pattern baldness).

As is so often the case, my lovely clients have been instrumental in scooting me up the aromatherapy ladder of learning and forcing me to find answers for the health and beauty problems they present me with. When one after another begged me to research hair growth as long as fifteen years ago, I was challenged to see what the precious oils could do. Out of that challenge came the hair growth kit and an even greater appreciation for the wonders of essential oils. It has reinforced my belief that nature's own plant medicines have the answer to many health and beauty issues. (See the Resource Guide.)

Essential oils not only nourish the hair and scalp; they help repel dirt. Some oils have properties that make them especially good for the hair and scalp, and it is these that I use in my practice and include in the recipes that follow.

Many people don't like the idea of using oil blends in their hair. They fear oil will leave the hair flat, limp, and greasy. This is not usually so, especially with the oils I recommend here. If you still feel hesitant about using these recipes, you can always just add a few drops of the recommended oils to your conditioner or shampoo, or give your scalp and hair an oil treatment an hour before shampooing.

As with any beauty concerns, you cannot separate healthy hair from a healthy body. To optimally nourish your hair, be sure you eat the healthy, rounded diet described in chapter 3. Fruits, vegetables, and fatty fish are key. If you can't quite manage the recommended daily and weekly allotments for the essential fatty acids, I suggest you supplement your diet with cod liver oil or flaxseed oil capsules daily. Also be sure you are getting sufficient vitamin B complex, plus a multimineral supplement with calcium, magnesium, silica, zinc, and potassium.

HATS OFF! HEAVENLY HAIR CONDITIONING OIL

Whatever your hair type, this is a wonderful conditioning treatment you can use up to 3 times a week. It is especially good for over-processed hair that color and/or perm treatments have stripped of all life.

    20 drops ylang-ylang essential oil
    10 drops lavender essential oil
    20 drops thyme essential oil
    20 drops chamomile essential oil
     1 ounce castor oil
     ½ ounce jojoba oil
     ½ ounce olive oil

Combine the essential oils with the base oils in a bottle. Before shampooing, massage 1 or 2 tablespoons of the blend into your hair and scalp using deep, circular movements. Wrap your hair with a hot, damp towel and relax for 20 minutes. Shampoo with a mild, organic shampoo.

Alternatively, you can pour 1 tablespoon of this oil directly into your favorite shampoo or conditioner and use as instructed.

As noted earlier, Missing Link powder, available through Designing Health (see Resource Guide) or at better health food stores, provides a marvelous combination of essential nutrients, vitamins, and minerals. It is easy to take and very effective for overall well-being. I find that 1 tablespoon daily is sufficient.

THE BODY

Many of my clients follow essential oil–based beauty preparations religiously on their face, then use harsh, detergent-type soap on their bodies. Your newly sensitized skin needs gentler, more moisturizing soaps for the body. You can use the following preparation whatever your skin type, wherever you are, with excellent results:

WAKE-UP CALL

- 30 drops lemongrass essential oil
- 30 drops lavender essential oil
- 30 drops rosemary essential oil
- 16 ounces unscented liquid castille soap (available in any health food or beauty supply store)

Add essential oils to castille soap and shake well. Store this mixture in a sturdy, recyclable plastic container. Use as an invigorating shower gel in the morning to start your day.

❧ BELOVED BODY SPLASH

This invigorating body splash is a feel-good, restorative treatment for use at any time. It is especially good for skin that has been sun damaged or exposed to extreme temperatures of any kind.

1   quart distilled water
1   orange peel
2   lemon peels
½   teaspoon thyme leaves
7   drops jasmine essential oil
3   tablespoons 100 proof vodka
8   ounces lavender water

Put distilled water in a clean glass jar. Add orange and lemon peels and thyme leaves. Place covered glass jar in a sunlit window, rotating the jar toward the sun, for 3 days. Each day, shake the jar to disperse the material. Meanwhile, put the jasmine oil in the vodka and leave in another quart bottle for 3 days.

After 3 days, strain out the citrus peels and thyme sediment and pour this distilled mixture into the quart bottle containing the jasmine and vodka mixture. Add the lavender water. Shake well, then rebottle in smaller, pretty containers. Store in a cool, dry place.

Use as an invigorating, skin-restoring after-bath splash, as a light cologne, or in cooling compresses after you've been out in the sun or at the beach.

SPECIAL SKIN PROBLEMS
Dermatitis/Eczema/Psoriasis

First, it is necessary to increase your dietary intake of essential fatty acids as described in chapter 2. Using essential oils externally as well makes for a double whammy that can create a whole new skin even for long-term sufferers of dermatitis, eczema, or psoriasis.

❧ SKIN BALANCING OIL

5	drops bergamot oil
20	drops carrot oil
10	drops lavender oil
10	drops juniper oil
15	drops sandalwood or myrrh oil
½	teaspoon camellia or rosa mosqueta oil
½	teaspoon grapeseed oil

Combine all ingredients in a 1-ounce bottle and mix well. Rub into affected areas, as well as surrounding tissue, at least twice daily.

Cornstarch and arrowroot powder can also help treat these skin conditions. Morning and night, take a cotton pad dusted with either of these powders and blot over affected areas after massaging in the aromatherapy blend.

CHAPTER 9

STRESS-BUSTING THERAPIES

~⌒

HAVE YOU EVER NOTICED HOW THOSE AT PEACE WITH THEMSELVES and the world look tranquil and rested, aglow with the loveliness of life, while those who are overstressed look nervous and haggard much of the time?

Modern life isn't always easy, and we all have our problems. For this reason, it is important to take control of our mental health and to make a conscious effort to relieve as much daily stress as we can. In this chapter, I provide techniques for doing just that—options that have worked wonders for both my clients and me for many years.

QUIET TIME

It is so important for our physical, mental, and spiritual health to just take the time—at least a few minutes every day—to do nothing. It doesn't matter whether this takes the form of day-dreaming, active meditation, or plain vegging out.

We inhabit a noisy, busy, stressful world. Everything is going full tilt: the radio, television, computer, chatter, traffic, and most of all, our very talkative and judgmental left brain. It just never seems to shut up, and with its judgments and activity come constant, sometimes inappropriate emotional responses. Thus, for some of us, life is an ongoing battle with many hidden dangers—often in our subconscious—just waiting to get to us.

It doesn't have to be this way. In fact, life is a constant battle only if we allow it to be. Regain some perspective by refusing to listen to the babble for a while. Turn off your left brain for a few minutes by giving yourself permission to be quiet, to listen to the silence, or to daydream. Some of us need help to get to this restful place and might need some soft music in a cozy, darkened room. Choose music that nourishes the soul, such as:

- nature-sound tapes with babbling brooks or wind sounds in the background
- soft classical music with harps or violins
- New Age tapes with chanting or piano melodies
- any other kind of music that eases your heart and does not

jar your lower abdomen (stomach problems *are* often the result of our mental and psychological state)

During this healing, quiet time, practice deep, slow breathing to release toxins, lift stress, and slow down your heartbeat. Taking quiet time outdoors, especially in the shade of a big, leafy tree, is always a good idea.

Need a helping hand for your quiet time? Try this calming oil:

❦ CALMING/MEDITATION OIL

- 20 drops cedarwood essential oil
- 20 drops sweet orange essential oil
- 20 drops frankincense essential oil
- 10 drops marjoram essential oil
- 1 ounce safflower oil

Combine all oils in a bottle. Shake to blend well. Sprinkle a few drops in a bowl of hot water and inhale during meditation. Place the bowl on a table near your head.

You can also use 2 tablespoons of this calming oil in a warm bath to wind down after a hectic or hard day. But be forewarned: You may find it difficult to leave the bath afterward!

Once quiet time becomes a regular part of your day, you will begin to feel more relaxed. You will also feel more alert and in tune with your environment. The happy result: a more peaceful, healthier, and somehow "wholer" you.

Do not spoil this balance by watching the news while eating your meals—a very stressful and unhealthy practice. Good digestion can only occur with slow, peaceful eating. (It is no wonder that most children with digestive problems come from homes where the stress level is extremely high; adults, too, can wreak the same havoc on their stomachs if they eat fast and in unpeaceable situations.)

NATURE WALKS AND EXERCISE

Even though we often forget it, we are a part of nature, and nature is a part of us. To reconnect with a benevolent nature, we must regularly do enjoyable things outdoors—going for long, meandering strolls around the park or in the countryside, or the more physically challenging activities of hiking, bike riding, mountain climbing, or roller blading. In any case, it's important to feel real air on our skin, breathe it into our lungs, and have it uplift our souls. If we really take in the scenery, the greens and blues will calm our spirits and rest our eyes. Take the time to admire the most beautiful woman of all—Mother Nature!

Exercise is another important building block of beauty and health. I personally prefer stretching, yoga, and dance, but aerobics have their place, too, if that is your choice. However, I don't recommend excessive weight lifting. Low weights are great for toning and definition, but I personally do not think bulked-up muscles are part of the picture of relaxed beauty and health.

Regardless of what forms of exercise you choose, the important thing is to make sure muscles and joints are stretched and lubricated to prevent injury; and to aim for strength and stamina, with increased suppleness overall.

MASSAGE THERAPY

Therapeutic massage given by a knowledgeable, caring professional is one of the best healing treatments that you can give yourself. Massage releases toxins from the cells, stimulates the circulation, passively exercises the muscles, boosts the immune system, and relaxes the brain, nerves, and emotions. When you add essential oils, the entire experience is amplified and the benefits multiplied. What's more, since essential oils are also beautifying to the skin, you will also look younger and more radiant.

I have been a licensed massage therapist for twenty years, and I find it truly gratifying to be able to help my clients find health and joy through aromatherapy. If you are interested in receiving a therapeutic massage, contact the massage schools or holistic centers in your area and have them recommend a therapist to you. If they do not offer aromatherapy massage, consider bringing your own aromatherapy blends. If you would like to become an aromatherapist yourself, consult the Resource Guide, or contact us at The Aromatherapy Institute in New York City.

POSITIVE THINKING/AFFIRMATIONS

Positive thinking and affirmations can also help to release stress from your life. It is very hard to be positive in the face of negative events, situations, and people, but sometimes that is the only remedy for long-standing personal stresses and challenges.

In metaphysics we say "act as if." What this means is that you try to ignore the obvious negatives of a situation by acting as if they aren't there. Constantly affirming the polar opposite of the negative eventually brings the obverse—the happy positive—into your life.

Here's a favorite affirmation:

I am a beautiful child of the Divine,
constantly receiving from and giving blessings to all things.

Start with this affirmation and go on from there. Your local bookstore will have several excellent books of affirmations from which to choose.

AROMA DIFFUSERS

There are some wonderful lamps and diffusers on the market. You can use these to put your favorite essential oils directly into your personal environment, be it your home, your office, or even your car. This is passive aromatherapy through inhalation, and it can be very effective indeed. You can decide whether your diffuser blends should be for:

- relaxing
- decongesting
- uplifting the spirit
- stimulating mind and body
- focusing
- meditating

A whole market has sprung up around the creation of products that help dispense essential oils into the air.

For ease and practicality, there are scent rings that you can place over lightbulbs with a few drops of your favorite scents added. However, be aware that essential oils do get very hot when placed on metal rings over lightbulbs. I have even heard of bulbs exploding as a result of the scent ring adhering to the bulb. If you use these rings, choose the ceramic type.

There are also aroma diffusers. Some of these diffusers are glass-tipped and utilize pure essential oils (without water). These work by pushing the aroma out into the air via an electrical motor.

My personal favorites, however, are the various models of aroma lamps available. I especially like the lamps that use hot water as the base for propelling scent into the air. My designer, Brett Slavin, has created beautiful glazed ceramic lamps in various styles and in serene colors; they are wonderful aroma diffusers and lovely to behold as well! Brett's lamps have a space at the base for a small candle and a container on top in which you can put water, plus a few drops of essential oils. When the candle is lit, the water heats up, pushing the oils into the air.

There are also a variety of small diffusers designed to hang on your car's windshield. Just be sure to use brain-stimulating oils, not the sedating ones!

Contact suppliers in the Resource Guide (at the end of this book) to find the aroma diffuser that best fits your needs.

Here are some of my favorite combinations for aroma diffusers. Put these mixtures into an aroma diffuser before lighting the candle or plugging it in. If your diffuser uses water, put water in the container before adding the oil blend.

❧ ENERGIZER/DECONGESTER

    10 drops peppermint essential oil
    10 drops pine essential oil
    10 drops lavender essential oil

❧ MEDITATION/CALMING BLEND

    10 drops patchouli essential oil
    10 drops nutmeg oil
    10 drops bergamot oil

FOCUSING/MENTAL CLARITY BLEND

10   drops basil essential oil
10   drops rosemary essential oil
10   drops birch essential oil
 5   drops pettigrain essential oil

THE BATH

One of the most pleasant and luxurious ways to use essential oils is to put them in the bath, turning your tub into a relaxing and restorative spa. An aromatherapy bath can work such wonders for your physical and emotional well-being that you will want to have one at least once or twice a week. Every day is even better. Bless yourself by doing just that!

Part of the fun and soul-fulfilling enjoyment of your bath comes with making your own aromatherapy bath blends. These should be selected to conform to your own special needs and whimsies. Below I describe some of my favorite combinations, all designed to heal your body while enhancing the aromatic pleasures and uplifting qualities of the essential oils themselves.

🦋 BODY AND SOUL APPRECIATION BLEND

10 drops Moroccan rose essential oil

5 drops lemon essential oil

6 drops nutmeg essential oil

4 drops patchouli essential oil

5 drops cedarwood essential oil

½ ounce rice bran oil, camellia oil, or grapeseed oil

Combine essential oils with the base oil in a bottle and blend well. Into a full, warm tub, pour 2 tablespoons of this blend and slowly immerse your deserving self. Relax in tub for at least 30 minutes. Since this is an extremely sedative mixture, you may want to have some melodic reminder to gently bring you back into your physical body. Be sure to keep the bathroom lights dim—or, even nicer, light some candles.

When you (reluctantly) emerge from this bath, you will feel so relaxed, languorous, and silky, you might well wonder where your worries went!

Please do not break the spell by stopping to scrub out the bath immediately. Either warn your family, or if you live alone, do it another day—it will wait!

Wrap yourself in clean towels or a robe and slip into bed for a nap. Or, if you bathe at night, just retire for the most relaxing, enchanting full night's sleep you've ever had. Pleasant dreams!

And now for an entirely different kind of bath.

❦ AFTER-SPORTS BATH

10	drops birch essential oil
5	drops geranium essential oil
5	drops clary sage essential oil
10	drops eucalyptus essential oil
5	drops lemongrass essential oil
½	ounce olive oil

Mix the essential oils with the olive oil in a bottle. Pour 2 tablespoons of this blend into a fairly hot bath. Stay in the tub for at least 20 minutes. This mixture is designed to restore strength and stamina to overworked muscles and nerves, and to release lactic acid and other deposits trapped with the body's tissues. It is also a decongesting and mind-clearing blend, so your lungs and sinuses will also be clearer after this bath.

This is a highly stimulating bath, so don't do it just before going to bed. A good time might be in the morning or late afternoon before dinner. Enjoy your newly refreshed day!

The next bath is actually based on a baby oil formula I devised. One day, when I was short on time, I used this in my bathwater and became almost instantly hooked. Regardless of what skin type you have, this is a wonderful, moisturizing, super-smelling bath oil for everyone.

❧ BABY LOVE BATH TREAT

2   ounces safflower oil
2   ounces olive oil
10   drops Roman chamomile essential oil
5   drops calendula essential oil
15   drops lavender essential oil

Combine all ingredients in a thick glass or treated plastic bottle. Shake to blend well. Add 2 tablespoons to your bath; enjoy the silky feel and residual moisturizing effect.

The following combination is designed to lessen the sometimes exhausting effects of jet lag and to bring you back to your new time zone sooner. I remember once having traveled nonstop for what seemed like a hundred years (a day filled with delayed planes, missed connections, and overbearing crowds). A full night's sleep and a cleansing shower did nothing to improve my mood, lift my tiredness, or make me feel like a human being again.

So I turned to my trusty travel oil blend and began the day anew with a full bath and this marvelous oil. When I emerged some fifteen minutes later, I felt as if I had released my old grumpy self down the drain, while the newly reborn me emerged, like Venus on the half shell! Try it, and you'll most certainly agree. Happy trails to you!

❦ THE ULTIMATE TRAVEL BATH OIL

10 drops basil essential oil

5 drops bergamot essential oil

20 drops orange essential oil

15 drops lavender essential oil

20 drops spearmint essential oil

½ ounce vegetable oil

Blend the essential oils with the vegetable oil in a bottle. Pour 2 table-spoons into a full, warm tub. Relax in this bath for about 20 minutes.

The next bath is designed to give a boost to your immune sys-tem while helping the circulation, kidneys, and pores do their job of identifying, collecting, and removing toxins from your body. It is also a warming antiviral blend, so any lurking fevers can be readily dissipated. If you're lucky, just one or two of these baths plus a good night's sleep might restore you to health. In any event, this health bath will quickly put you on the road to recovery and have you feeling much better right away.

Finally, the last bath is one of my all-time favorite de-stressors, an all-purpose herbal beauty oil so versatile it might have gone anywhere in the book. Use this creamy, fragrant oil as a massage or bath oil or as a luxurious, lasting face moisturizer, or add some to your body lotion or hot-oil hair-conditioning treatment.

🦋 THE GET HEALTHY BATH (OR "HELP! I'M COMING DOWN WITH SOMETHING . . .")

10 drops ginger essential oil
5 drops blue chamomile essential oil
5 drops geranium essential oil
10 drops benzoin or Peru balsam essential oil
½ ounce olive oil

Combine the essential oils with the olive oil in a bottle and mix well. Pour 2 tablespoons into a fairly hot bath and relax for at least 30 minutes.

🦋 YELLOW PEACE

1 handful fresh white rose petals
½ handful fresh pink rose petals
Skin from 1 cucumber
12 ounces pure virgin olive oil
4 ounces safflower oil
6 drops rose essential oil

Combine all ingredients in a 16-ounce glass mason jar and place on a sunny windowsill, rotating frequently for 3 days. After the third day, remove the cucumber skin and some of the rose petals. Leave a few of the petals in for beauty's sake.

CHAPTER 10

A SHORT GUIDE TO THE ESSENTIAL OILS

AROMATHERAPY IS THE SCIENCE AND USAGE OF ESSENTIAL OILS. As explained in chapter 1, oils are made up of incredibly complex chemical components named terpenes.

Of the billions of plant species existing on Earth, a small fraction contribute scented and medicinal plants, and although only sixteen to twenty botanical families are represented in aromatherapy, some families donate multiple members—the mint and carrot families, for example.

In *Essential Beauty*, we have featured only a few of the one hundred or so essential oils used in aromatherapy, but they cover a variety of plants from thirteen botanical families.

ESSENTIAL OIL FAMILIES
Annonaceae

Ylang-ylang is the essential oil member of this family most commonly used in aromatherapy. A similar oil, cananga, is the end result of extraction of the flower of a slightly different cousin, *Cananga odorata*. Ylang-ylang is *Cananga odorata genuina*.

This botanical family is found mainly in the tropics, with cananga contributing the only sweet-scented essential oil, so far as we now know. Other members also produce soft, sweet, dessert-like fruits found only in the tropics, like custard apple (annona) and sweetsop (a cousin to guanabana). Sweetsop has been described as "vanilla ice cream from the tree," and that description is right on. Delectable!

Burseraceae

Both frankincense and myrrh belong to this family, as do opopanax and elemi. Family members produce gummy resins that have been used all over the world since ancient times for skin care, as expectorants to remove mucus from the respiratory tracts, and in religious services.

Compositae

This is the ubiquitous daisy family, a prolific and generous group. We mainly use chamomile in aromatherapy, but marigold (or calendula) is also a valuable healing oil, as are arnica, tagetes, and helichrysum.

The Compositae are very popular in herbology; for example, echinacea, elecampane, chicory, dandelion, boneset, yarrow, tagetes, helichrysum, and tarragon are all members of the daisy family. We also get important dietary oils from this family, such as safflower, sunflower, and canola (rapeseed).

Cupressaceae

Cypress, cedarwood, and juniper are the most famous members of the aromatherapy cast. They each donate essential oils from different areas of the plant. Cypress oil comes from the leaves, cedarwood oil from the wood, and juniper oil from the berry but also occasionally from the leaves.

In esoterica, we see them as energetically representing different centers of the body—cypress, the head; juniper, the middle; and cedarwood, the base.

Geraniaceae

The geranium family gives us the lovely, decoratively scented pelargoniums and our own summertime window box of geraniums.

Geranium essential oil comes from herb Robert *(Geranium robertianum)*, a shrubby plant native to South Africa and found in many other places. Sometimes called cranesbill, Algerian bourbon, or Moroccan geranium, all have been used throughout history as styptics (wound healers). A styptic is an agent that aids the clotting mechanism of the blood.

Geranium is also an extremely effective circulation booster or rubefacient (skin reddener) that brings warmth to the peripheral areas. Thus it is a wonderful oil to use during cold weather, especially on the feet and hands.

Occasionally, people are allergic to geranium oil on the face and can break out in red rashes. This is because of the heating quality of the oil. If you remember to mix this oil with other cooler ones such as lavender or pine, that problem should be averted.

Geraniol, a large component of geranium oil, is found in all essential oils in lesser amounts. As a result, it could be truthfully stated that all essential oils are good for the circulation because of their geraniol content, but geranium has an edge, because it has the most.

Labiatae
(Mint Family)

The packhorses of the medicinal and flavoring herb family! This family contains thousands of members, including such dissimilar relatives as patchouli, mint, bergamot (Oswego tea), basil, melissa, and motherwort.

Of course, some people only recognize peppermint and spearmint as mints, but they are just two of the many members donating essential oils to aromatherapy. In addition to those mentioned above, other members include lavender, marjoram, hyssop, pennyroyal, rosemary, sage, and thyme.

Mints all work to decongest the sinuses and respiratory tracts. They also clean out the digestive tract and tone and balance the liver and gallbladder. The vast majority of mints are refrigerants (or coolants) to the skin.

Myrtaceae
(Myrtle Family)

Found all over the world, this family was named for the European myrtle but includes essential oil plant members like bay (there is also a bay laurel), allspice, clove, eucalyptus, nutmeg, and tea tree.

These scented plants are all big trees with shiny leaves and a pungent aroma. They are very similar to another large-tree/pungent-scented family—Lauraceae (the laurel family), with members such as sassafras, rosewood, and cinnamon bay. In fact, these two families have been frequently confused over the ages.

Myrtaceae members are strongly antiseptic and antiviral, and work especially well with lung and digestive tract problems. Interesting fact: The tropical fruit guava is also a member of the Myrtaceae family.

Oleaceae
(Olive Family)

Olive oil is a favorite dietary oil of mine, but I also use it as a carrier oil for hair conditioning blends and digestive tract blends.

Jasmine, its cousin, is another favorite. I love its sweet, musty aroma. Jasmine oil has many terpenes in common with other flowers, such as jasmone, neroli, geraniol, and linalool.

The jasmine used in aromatherapy comes from the *Jasminum officinale*, *grandiflorum*, and *sambac* species. It does not, as some people think, come from the Carolina jasmine or yellow jessamine, which is from a totally different family (the poisonous Loganiaceae).

Rosaceae

The rose family is kin to a huge variety of plants—about five thousand members—all having in common pretty flowers and sweet gourmet fruits, such as peaches, apricots, strawberries, black cherries, blackberries, and almonds.

We get essential oils from the white or pink roses, not the more flamboyantly colored ones. Major rose oil–producing countries include France, Bulgaria, Morocco, Turkey, Italy, and China. Rose oil contains, among other things, geraniol, neroli, and citronella. Roses grown in hot, sunshiny places like Morocco and the tropics produce a sweeter-smelling oil than roses grown in more northern countries.

Rutaceae

A very innocuous-looking shrub has given its name to the flamboyant, flirtatious citrus family. In fact, rue has a strong European history relating it to poisons and witchcraft.

In aromatherapy, the citrus family members donate their essential oils through their peels, leaves, or flowers. For example: bergamot, lemon, lime, mandarin, sweet and bitter orange, tangerine (peels), neroli (flowers), and pettigrain (leaves and young shoots).

These citruses certainly bring warmth, sunshine, and joy into whatever blends they are part of, and all of them are skin-friendly. To avoid photosensitivity, be sure to combine with coolants like lavender, resins like benzoin, or woods like cedarwood and sandalwood.

Santalaceae
(Sandalwood Family)

This tree is native to India and Southeast Asia and has a distinctive bittersweet/woodsy tone. There are different plants called sandalwood or saunderswood, but the one valued in aromatherapy for its essential oil comes from the Mysore region of India; thus, it is known as Mysore sandalwood.

Styracaceae

A resinous family that includes gum benzoin *(Styrax benzoin)* and *S. tokinensis*. Family members are huge trees (up to 120 feet high) with white blossoms. The resin is extracted by incision in the bark. These trees are native to tropical Asia. The resins are heavily vanillin, have cinnamic notes, and have traditionally been used to heal sores and wounds and for skin care and lung cleansing.

A similar family, Storax, whose members include amber, American storax, and liquidambar, exudes a similarly scented and used resin but is native to America. Botanists have constantly interchanged the two families because of their similarities.

Umbelliferae
(Carrot Family)

Another varied and plentiful family with members worldwide, Umbelliferae grows wild and sometimes looks similar to the Compositae. Its essential oil family members include anise, angelica, carrot, coriander, fennel, parsley, and caraway, among others. These members are active digestive aids and diuretics, and are quite skin-friendly. They all also have a vague similarity in aroma.

THE ESSENTIAL OILS

All essential oils should be diluted for application on the skin. The general rule of thumb for adults is 4 drops essential oil(s) to 1 tablespoon carrier oil and 1 drop essential oil(s) per tablespoon for children. I prefer to use vegetable oil as a carrier instead of petroleum-based oils. My favorite vegetable oil is safflower. It has very little scent, so it won't interfere with the aroma of the essential oils, it is light and absorbable, and it does not stain fabrics as much as other vegetable oils.

Another important point is that aromatherapists always combine three to five essential oils in blends because that is the most effective and safest way to use them. By using a blend of essential oils, the negative effects of overabsorption of any one chemical component found in a particular oil can be mitigated. Using just one essential oil continuously can lead to toxic reactions in the body.

Bay Myrtle
(Myrtaceae)

The essential oil of leaves of the bay myrtle has a vanilla-like substance called eugenol. This is used to make commercial vanilla and is also used in many products as a digestive aid. Eugenol also has an anti-inflammatory effect on the skin. Bay is excellent for oily or acne-prone skin, as well as for men's skin, because of its astringent properties. It is a light, cooling oil that is also wonderful to use in hot weather as a splash.

Years ago, bay was popularized as a tropical splash called bay rum. Bay is not to be used alone for dry or sensitive skin.

Benzoin
(Styracaceae)

This is a gummy, resinous oil, redolent of vanilla, chocolate, and molasses, which is excellent for all skin types. I adore this oil but find it very frustrating to work with in blends. It refuses to mix with most other essential oils and quickly sinks to the bottom of the blend. It sometimes does that in creams, too, or it just separates and striates the cream, with pinkish/amber stripes.

Don't let these minor inconveniences stop you from using benzoin. Benzoin is extremely friendly for all skin types. Just remember to reshake the mixture before applying the oil to your skin to bring the benzoin to the top.

Bergamot
(Rutaceae)

Bergamot is an orange oil that has been used mostly in cosmetics rather than in food. It is used, however, in Earl Grey tea and is responsible for the tea's perfumy aroma. Bergamot oil has gotten a bad rap as a possible skin cancer agent, even though a leading authority, E. Guenther, in his multivolume *Essential Oils,* reported that when he tested this oil, he found that the skin became more photosensitive only when bergamot oil was mixed with alcohol.

Bergamot is remarkably skin-friendly. It softens the skin, smoothes and evens out skin tone, and stimulates the release of melanin in the skin cells. Melanin is a brown pigment that the skin produces as a result of exposure to the sun, to help screen out the harmful rays of the sun. Thus, melanin—and bergamot without the alcohol—is actually a protective agent.

Carrot Seed
(Umbelliferae)

Carrot seed oil is an orange-colored kerosene-smelling oil that the skin adores. The carotene in this oil is converted into vitamin A, which has a speedy, regenerating action on the skin.

I've used this oil on all skin types—babies to seniors—and the result is always the same: skin that is supple and soft. As such, carrot seed is especially effective for leathery, dehydrated, wrinkled, and sun-damaged skins. Its potent smell can be somewhat neutralized by mixing it with floral oils, such as rose or jasmine. Better still, learn to love carrot seed's smell. It's indicative of this oil's wonderful beautifying prowess!

Cedarwood
(Cupressaceae)

This immense, ancient tree has inspired a whole series of mythologies around the world. Cedarwood symbolizes strength, longevity, spirituality, and/or immortality.

The woody-smelling oil is a wonderful addition to men's skin-care products and is especially good for oily or acne-prone skin types. Cedarwood is also very effective for reducing the thickened, open-pored congestion that some skin develops over time, and the refining action is greatly aided by combining it with lemon or lime oil.

Cedarwood's smell may initially prove too strong to your liking, but give it a chance. By regularly massaging it into your skin, you will notice its relaxing, soothing effect on your entire nervous system.

Chamomile
(Compositae)

Roman and especially blue chamomile are the darlings of the skin-care industry. Azulene, a blue-green chemical that is fabulous in treating broken capillaries and sensitive skin, is a major component of the chamomiles, notably the blue variety.

Chamomile is good for all skin types—from cradle to grave—and the essential oil has a very soothing, cooling effect on the nerves and skin. Blue chamomile has been more popular because of its color, which is a beautiful addition to creams and lotions. It is very comforting and soothing to apply a pale blue cream to the skin, don't you think? However, the apple-scented Roman chamomile is fast gaining ground and is my favorite of the two because of its uplifting aroma.

Cypress
(Cupressaceae)

The essential oil comes from the leaves of this wonderful tree. Incredibly sharp smelling, it is definitely an acquired taste! What I like best about cypress is its muscle-firming quality. It is very effective in a face and neck combination and also for cellulite and other body-toning treatments.

Cypress is good for all complexion types. However, you will have to soften its harsh smell with gentler essential oils like rose, lavender, or orange.

Frankincense
(Burseraceae)

This shrubby bush originated in Somalia, Ethiopia, and Yemen and has been revered since ancient days as both a holy oil and a beauty potion. In fact, it has long been associated with the Queen of Sheba's beauty routines. Because of the lure of frankincense, several important trade routes were established in the ancient world when conquering nations wanted this oil (along with its cousin myrrh).

The frankincense plant thrives in adverse desert conditions. Its oil is actually a resin that oozes out of slashes or cuts made in the stems or bark. This sweet-smelling resin is a wonderful moisturizer. It is also a humectant; its oil traps moisture in the skin cells, leaving the skin's surface smooth and plumped out.

Thus, frankincense is especially good for dry, mature, and/or weathered skins, but it can also be used to excellent effect on normal and combination skin types.

Frankincense is also a natural decongestant that is relaxing to the nerves and to the brain. For this reason, it is possible to achieve a very uplifting (both mentally and physically) facial when this oil is part of the blend.

You may also have seen frankincense in its other form—beige-colored beads with a powdery surface called "frankincense tears," commonly used in potpourris. If you were to put these tears in oil, they would reliquefy.

Geranium
(Geraniaceae)

This wildflower is called herb Robert in some countries. The oil itself smells rather like a spicy, lemony rose; typically, it provokes strong reactions of either love or hate. See page 153 for more information about geranium essential oil.

Grapefruit
(Rutaceae)

Like all citrus, grapefruit makes and stores essential oils in the outer peel of the fruit's skin. I love this essential oil and its lovely, fruity smell.

Grapefruit is great for a full range of skin types. It works wonders against cellulite and fluid retention. Grapefruit is a tremendous circulation booster. As well, it is a warming oil that immediately reddens the skin (in technical terms, a rubefacient) and makes skin supple. Grapefruit is lovely in men's facial blends, for combination skins, and to counteract extremely dry skin.

Jasmine
(Oleaceae)

This very sweet, sultry flower belongs in formulas designed to regenerate skin cells, eliminate couperose, and firm muscle tone. Whenever I'm demonstrating my facial technique, I try (to the fullest extent possible) to include jasmine or other floral oils in my blends, because the results they provide are so spectacular.

One of my clients loved jasmine so much that she wanted to use this oil everywhere on her body. She placed a jasmine blend directly on some reddened stretch marks on her thighs, and voilà, the unsightly areas disappeared in just a few days.

Juniper Berry
(Cupressaceae)

Juniper is a wonderful combination fruity/woodsy oil. Although terrific for many skin problems, juniper is best used for the legs and tummy.

Juniper is also good as a diuretic oil and, like its cousin cypress, is excellent for cellulite and muscle-toning needs.

Although juniper smells like its fermented liquor (gin), juniper oil can be massaged into the liver area to help counteract the adverse effects of alcohol consumption.

I often use juniper oil as my personal antiperspirant/deodorant of choice.

Lavender
(Labiatae)

Lavender, which gets its name from the Latin root word *lavare* (to wash), has long been associated with the scent of freshly washed clothes and sheets, and also epitomizes clean, healthy, just-washed skin.

Lavender oil is certainly one of the best-known oils in all of aromatherapy. Its cool, minty aroma is just wonderful for most complexion needs and is also very good for hair care and hair regrowth. Because it is a refrigerant (cooling) oil, it is also comfortable in hot weather. In any season, lavender water is a wonderfully refreshing toner for many skin types.

Among its many other virtues, lavender has a deserved reputation as a sleep oil. This works for 90 percent of the people who try it. Another 10 percent will find that it has the opposite effect—it keeps them awake! They are responding to the more stimulating, complex notes of the French lavender and might do better with the softer English lavender.

Myrrh
(Burseraceae)

A relative of frankincense, this resinous oil has traditionally been used as the yin to frankincense's yang. However, myrrh is a darker, stronger-smelling oil than frankincense. It is very efficacious as an emollient for dehydrated, leathery, or aging skin.

A little bit of myrrh goes a long way. I have found that myrrh oil is too heavy for young or oily skins. However, I have friends from the Middle East and Northeast Africa who have used myrrh oil on their skins since childhood—and their skins love it. I think it is all a matter of what you are used to.

Myrrh is, of course, also famous as a meditation oil used in religious and spiritual rituals, along with its cousin frankincense.

Neroli (Orange Blossom)
(Rutaceae)

Truly the queen of all skin-care oils, neroli *(Citrus aurantium)* has a beautiful citrus blossom scent, and is a beautifier for all types of skin, from babies to seniors. When properly used, neroli truly makes the face bloom like a flower.

Until quite recently, many European brides always carried a bouquet of orange blossoms at their weddings. This was a symbol of beauty, happiness, and fertility. In fact, in esoterica, neroli is called "mantrap" because it is said to put a man in a marrying mood!

Pure neroli essential oil is extremely expensive, just like jasmine and rose; but, as is the case with the others, a few drops will do wonders in a skin-care blend.

Patchouli
(Labiatae)

This musty hippie favorite is a member of the fresh-smelling mint family; it's the kind of aroma people either love or hate.

To be honest, I am both intrigued and put off by patchouli's marijuana-like aroma, but I can certainly attest to its marvelous and beneficial therapeutic effects. It is also a skin-friendly oil that's great for circulation problems such as cellulite and fluid retention. Other folks are intrigued by patchouli, too. In fact, one major company specializing in fabric softeners recently cornered the market on patchouli, nearly depleting the resources for aromatherapists.

Rose
(Rosaceae)

The delicate soft petals of the rose have represented the epitome of beauty throughout history.

Rose oil comes mainly from two sources, damask rose (*Rosa damascena*) and *Rosa centifolia*, and is sold as Bulgarian Rose and

Moroccan Rose. Both rose oils smell totally different, but they both act beautifully on the skin.

I like to use rose oil for baby and infant care, and for thin, dry skin, although it is excellent for virtually every skin type. After an aromatherapy-based facial that includes rose oil, one's skin should feel as soft and smooth as a baby's bottom and look like a rose petal.

Rosemary
(Labiatae)

Yet another member of the hardworking mint family, rosemary is a prickly, feisty herb with a camphorated eucalyptus smell. It has a very long association with hair growth and memory, but this oil is also superlative in dislodging cysts under the skin and in combating fluid retention.

Rosemary is also a wonderful antidote to saggy skin and fatty deposits. I once had a client with virtually no muscle tone in her tummy; she never exercised and thus had loose, flabby flesh throughout the abdomen area. She did, however, come to me for a weekly massage in hopes of helping firm up her tummy. I made this woman a rosemary blend and asked her to massage it into her tummy region every day while she was lying on the couch watching television. She did so, and the results were clearly visible after only a few weeks. Had she exercised, the change would have been even more spectacular.

Clary Sage
(Lamiaceae, Labiatae)

Yet another mint, sage also has a musty but cool aroma that at first whiff seems masculine. However, given its high estrogen content, sage is actually a feminine oil that balances hormones and emotions splendidly.

Sage has long been used for mental clarity and hair growth. In the Southwest region of this country, burning sage to remove negativity is a Native American tradition that has spread to many other parts of the world.

Sage oil is especially good for muscle tone and strength, against cellulite, and to improve circulation problems. Thus, I include sage in sports blends to help overworked muscles release the lactic acid that might have built up. Similarly, sage is an excellent bruise and wound healer.

Sandalwood
(Santalaceae)

One of the scents strongly identified with India, sandalwood oil has a distinctive, resinous/woodsy smell that sets some people completely at ease, while utterly agitating others.

Sandalwood is very popular in perfumery and skin-care products. It is also used for meditation and essential sleep blends. Furthermore, sandalwood is a terrific lubricant and is friendly to all skin types. It is also extremely soothing to the nerves and helps balance the circulation.

Even though I myself am not overly fond of sandalwood's scent, I admire its effectiveness in complexion and body care. By judiciously combining it with what I find to be far pleasanter oils, I use it quite often myself and in blends for my clients.

Ylang-Ylang
(Annonaceae)

The "flower of flowers" of Malaysia, syrupy-sweet ylang-ylang oil combines the beauty of a blossom with the aftertaste of cough syrup in its unique aroma. Pronounced *eelang-eelang,* this flower and its oil bring a long association of joy and aphrodisia to our cynical, overly busy world.

A friend of mine, who has an aromatherapy shop in Port-of-Spain, Trinidad, says that his blend of ylang-ylang and patchouli flies off the shelves because both men and women love it and wear it as a primary body scent. I myself use ylang-ylang for all complexion types to help maintain youth and beauty of the cells. What's more, it is a wonderful way to soothe hyperstressed types as well as those with average levels of modern-day stress.

Resource Guide

The following resource guide is a valuable tool for persons interested in obtaining products, information, and other supplies.

The Aromatherapy Institute
P.O. Box 909
New York, NY 10274-2909
Tel: (212) 545-0229
Fax: (212) 545-1335
www.escentiallyyours.com

Offers a 200-hour diploma program consisting of various modules of study. On completion, you will be a fully trained aromatherapist. Also offers a one-on-one apprentice training program, certificate programs, and visiting programs.

Aromatic Thymes (magazine)
P.O. Box 3279
N. Las Vegas, NV 89036
Tel: (877) 355-1168 (toll free)
Fax: (702) 437-4547
Athymes@aol.com

A wonderful magazine for aromatherapy information.

Designing Health
28310 Avenue Crocker, Unit G
Valencia, CA 91355
Tel: 1-800-774-7387
www.designinghealth.com

Sells Missing Link powder, a synergistic blend of whole and super foods developed by Drs. Udo Erasmus and Robert Collett.

E-Scentially Yours
P.O. Box 909
New York, NY 10274-0909
Tel: (212) 545-0229 or 1-800-927-5402 (orders only)
Fax: (212) 545-1335
www.escentiallyyours.com

Essential oils, aromatherapy blends and products, aroma lamps, books, charts, gift baskets, hair growth kit, and other supplies.

The Essential Oil Company
1719 SE Umatilla
Portland, OR 97202
http://essentialoil.com
Tel: 1-800-729-5912
Fax: 1-800-825-2985

Essential oils, massage oils, aromatherapy and perfume materials, books, and glassware.

Medicine Flower, Inc.
P.O. Box 1127
Corvallis, OR 97339
Orders: 1-800-787-3645
Tel: (541) 745-3055
Fax: (541) 745-3056
www.medicineflower.com

Essential oils, carrier oils, candles, perfume oils, lotions, bottles, droppers, and packaging.

Most Essential
wendymost@worldnet.att.net

Bath and body oils.

Jeanne Rose
Aromatherapy Educator
219 Carl Street
San Francisco, CA 94117
Tel: (415) 564-6785 or (415) 564-6799

Classes arranged in different locations.

Kitty's Soap
Bronx, NY 10469
(718) 655-4850

Handmade essential oils, soaps, spritzers for care and home,
and handmade skin creams.

Zenith Supplies, Inc.
6300 Roosevelt Way NE
Seattle, WA 98115
Tel: 1-800-735-7217
Fax: (206) 525-3703
www.zenithsupplies.com

Aromatherapy oils and products.

BIBLIOGRAPHY

⸜⸝

Balick, Michael J., and Paul Alan Cox. *Plants, People & Culture. The Science of Ethnobotany.* New York: Scientific American Library, 1996.

Beckstrom-Sternberg, Stephen M., and James A. Duke. *CRC Handbook of Medicinal Mints.* Boca Raton, Fla.: CRC Press, Inc., 1996.

Bisset, Norman Grainger, ed., and Max Wichtl. *Herbal Drugs and Phytopharmaceuticals.* Boca Raton, Fla.: CRC Press, Inc., 1994.

Duke, James A. *The Green Pharmacy.* Emmaus, Pa.: Rodale Press, 1997.

Gallant, Ann. *Principles and Techniques for the Beauty Specialist,* 2d ed. Cheltenham, England: Stanley Thornes Ltd., 1980.

Gattefossé, René-Maurice. *Gattefossé's Aromatherapy,* edited by Robert Tisserand. Saffron Walden, England: C. W. Daniel Company, 1993.

Leung, Albert Y., and Steven Foster. *Encyclopedia of Common Natural Ingredients Used in Food, Drugs and Cosmetics.* New York: John Wiley & Sons, Inc., 1996.

List, P. H., and P. C. Schmidt. *Phytopharmaceutical Technology.* Boca Raton, Fla.: CRC Press, Inc., 1989.

Roebuck, Anne. *Aroma-Spa Therapy.* Toronto: Anessence, 1995.

Rose, Jeanne. *Kitchen Cosmetics.* San Francisco: Self-published, 1978.

——. *The World of Aromatherapy.* Berkeley, Calif.: Frog Ltd., 1996.

Schultes, Richard Evans, ed. *Medicines from the Earth.* Maidenhead, England: McGraw-Hill Book Co., 1983.

Tisserand, Robert. *Aromatherapy for Everyone.* London: Penguin Books, 1988.

BOOKS FOR FURTHER READING

Ackerman, Diane. *A Natural History of the Senses.* New York: Random House, 1990.

Arvigo, Rosita, and Michael Balick. *Rainforest Remedies: One Hundred Healing Herbs of Belize.* Twin Lakes, Wis.: Lotus Press, 1993.

Betty, Patricia. *Aromatherapy: A Personal Journey Through Your Senses.* New York: Carnegie Press, 1994.

Damian, Peter and Kate. *Aromatherapy Scent and Psyche.* Rochester, Vt.: Healing Arts Press, 1995.

Garland, Sarah. *The Complete Book of Herbs and Spices.* New York: Viking Press, 1979.

Magic and Medicine of Plants. Purchase, N.Y.: Reader's Digest Press, 1993.

Rose, Jeanne. *375 Essential Oils and Hydrosols.* Berkeley, Calif.: Frog Ltd., 1999.

INDEX

('I' INDICATES AN ILLUSTRATION, 'T' INDICATES A TABLE)

"Pat Betty's aromatherapy has been part of the Power of Herbs lecture series at The New York Botanical Garden for over four years. Her expertise in the field is displayed in both her enthusiasm and her ability to actually demonstrate this healing art."

—Erica Kipp, Manager, Plant Research Lab, The New York Botanical Garden

"Pat Betty helped me in my personal quest to know more about aromatherapy and acted as a mentor in this journey."

—Maureen Ressler, Training Director, Elizabeth Arden Salons

"Pat Betty has been actively involved in aromatherapy in New York City for many years. She is a natural perfumer and describes [essential oils] in her own unique, trademark way."

—*The Aromatic Thymes*

"Aromatherapy skin care really works. Pat Betty is an expert with years of experience."

—Anne Roebuck, author of *Aroma Spa-Therapy*

In *Essential Beauty*, Patricia Betty, one of America's foremost aromatherapists, shares her internationally renowned beauty formulas, all derived from nature's own essential oils. Featuring dozens of unique, easy recipes for moisturizers, exfoliators, toners, and other natural treatments, this book also offers Betty's exclusive natural ~~holistic alternatives to packaged cosmet-~~ ics, and food ~~and beauty~~. *Essential Beauty* is a guide for anyone who wants to experience the life-affirming joy of nature's essential oils.

Patricia Betty is the owner of E-scentially Yours aromatherapy center in New York City. A staff member of The New York Botanical Garden, she has served as a consultant to Elizabeth Arden and other companies.

David Andrusia is the author of twelve books, including *Branding Yourself, Gentle Healing for Your Baby and Child,* and *The Perfect Pitch.* A graduate of Columbia University, the Sorbonne, and the Annenberg School for Communications, he lives in Los Angeles and New York.

COVER DESIGN BY LAURIE YOUNG
PHOTOGRAPH BY FPG / © TELEGRAPH COLOUR LIBRARY 1997

US $16.95 / CAN $24.95

ISBN 0-658-00280-5

51695>

9 780658 002809